PREVENT THIS

**Dedicated to Raphael Cabrera
and
The Institute of Integrative Nutrition
for helping me find my voice.**

**Cindy Fuchser RN, BSN, CCRN
Health Coach**

Prevent This

A Simple Guide to Beat Disease

About the Author

Cindy Fuchser was 10 years old when she watched a 60 Minutes segment about reversing cardiovascular disease with diet and lifestyle modifications. Many years later, working as a critical care nurse caring for cardiovascular-diseased patients and those with numerous other preventable conditions, it became apparent to Cindy that western-trained physicians were not informing patients about behaviors and foods detrimental to health. What she learned was that today's healthcare system perpetuates disease by ignoring safe and inexpensive health-saving strategies while recommending dangerous procedures and prescribing ineffective drugs wrought with adverse side effects.

Cindy received her Bachelor of Science degree in Nursing from San Diego State University and has been certified as a Critical Care RN for more than 20 consecutive years by the American Association of Critical Care Nurses. Her disappointment in our healthcare delivery system led her to the Institute of Integrative Nutrition, where she obtained her Certification as a Health and Wellness Coach.

Cindy was first published in the Journal of Gluten Sensitivity after passionately writing, "The Gluten Free Diet Is Not Just Another Fad Diet," a response to inaccurate health information delivered by a registered dietitian at the hospital where she worked. Because Cindy knows how devastating and costly "chronic" illness is and how easy it can be to avoid if you make an effort, she has written this book to help you make health a priority in your life.

Learn more about Cindy and her healthy lifestyle at bodysavior.com.

Foreword

Whether you've decided you want to live life in good health or you're just tired of taking prescription medication, you've done the right thing by picking up this book.

My friend Cindy Fuchser, the author of this book, is a registered nurse. I've known Cindy for over a decade. She is dedicated and passionate about the good health and well-being of others, and she is very concerned about the needless suffering experienced by people around the world because of their diet and lifestyle choices. She understands better than most that making smarter choices can prevent many health conditions, and she questions why doctors are so quick to prescribe costly medicine rather than healthy food and exercise.

Over the years, I've noticed a deficit of knowledge in the medical community regarding natural disease prevention methods. Cindy has noticed it too and speaks up in support of accurate health information for patients and the community, searching far and wide to gather information about ancient wisdom and healing modalities.

With the Hippocratic approach of "let food be thy medicine and medicine be thy food," she practices what she preaches. Cindy's thirst for knowledge about all things healthy is on her mind on and off the hospital floor. She feels it's her responsibility to help change old healthcare methods and replace them with a more natural approach through diet and lifestyle.

The information she provides in this short and easy-to-read book will help both men and women discover there are other ways besides pharmaceuticals and surgeries to enhance and lengthen our lives. Her vision is not just for us to live long, but to live healthy as long as we live. Cindy seamlessly moves from what's making us sick to what steps we can take to change our health future for the better. She believes regeneration is possible at any age. I've personally experienced this transformation, so I know her words are true. Science has proven that genes play only a small part in how well and long we live, which means the rest is up to us. This is very empowering once you learn what you can do to improve your health.

I believe what Cindy most wants people to learn from this book is that serious illness can be avoided with just a few simple changes. People who lack energy can regain it. Prescriptions don't have to be life sentences. "Chronic" illnesses can be cured and ultimately avoided. Patients can heal themselves. We have the power to control our own health — without prescription drugs or surgery.

Today's fast foods and processed foods are

laced with hormones, antibiotics, steroids, pesticides, and artificial colors and flavorings. Rancid fats from frying and baking, along with poor cooking methods, are making our food unhealthy to consume. So, what to do? The answers in this book will strike a cord with anyone of any age. You will not feel restricted by changing your diet, but you will discover a newfound enjoyment of fresh foods that can provide you and your loved ones with energy and good health.

Most people my age are expected to have "age-related diseases." Several years ago, at age 69, I received cholesterol and blood pressure prescriptions from my doctor. I didn't want to take the medications, so I changed my diet instead. Changing my diet reduced my cholesterol and blood pressure and stopped arthritis in its tracks, too. Today I am vital, healthy, and prescription-free at age 76.

In this book, Cindy gives you a glimpse of what your own health future can be with just a little knowledge and some simple changes. If your health is important to you, this book is vitally important to read.

Mimi Kirk

Founder of youngonrawfood.com
Best-selling author of Live Raw, Live Raw Around the World, and The Ultimate Book of Modern Juicing
International speaker

Plant-based chef
Health coach and consultant

Prevent This
A Simple Guide to Beat Disease

Introduction

Caring for the sick and dying over the last 25 years as a critical care nurse has provided me an up-close view of what it's like to be chronically ill in the United States. Americans suffer from a multitude of "chronic," debilitating conditions years before we take our last breath. This ill state of health negatively impacts our minds and bodies and carves a giant dent in our pocketbooks. As a nation, we can't afford modern medicine. Too many of us are sick, and it comes at too high of a price in terms of both financial cost and human suffering.

Especially disturbing is the dramatic decline in the ages of my patients since I began nursing in 1988. At that time, the age of my critically ill patients was typically 65 to 80 and older. Now it seems that over one-half the patient population at Palomar Medical Center critical care unit, where I've worked for the last 18 years, is under 65.

My patients usually have between three and 10 diagnosis; hypertension, obesity, diabetes, coronary artery disease, congestive heart failure, chronic obstructive pulmonary disease (COPD), hyperlipidemia (more recently dyslipidemia), gastric esophageal reflux disease (GERD), peripheral vascular disease, and hypothyroidism are the most prevalent. In the last several years, I've noticed depression and the prescribing of

Antidepressants to the chronically ill is a growing trend. This souring of bodily functions at the end (or middle) of life is bad enough, but compound that with spending your life's savings on medical care, and it's easy to see why the chronically ill get depressed.

My personal inquiry into the cause and prevention of disease has led me to the conclusion that the cause of heart disease and depression are one and the same, and both are easily preventable. The same is true for most disease.

The suffering and loss that results from illness is particularly hard for me to swallow, because I understand how simple and inexpensive real health care can be and how forgiving the human body can be when it is provided with what it needs. You need not accept a diagnosis of illness as if it is bad weather and out of your control. As long as you are not six feet under, you have the power every day to make choices that improve your health; you can even eliminate so-called "chronic" ailments. The body is ever-changing; it replaces nearly 100 percent of its cells every three to six months, and this is what gives you the opportunity to achieve optimum health even if you've temporarily lost it.

My personal ongoing health journey began in grade school when I routinely witnessed an elderly neighbor jog up and down the street, probably no more than a mile or so. She was obviously older than my mom, close to my grandmother's age, yet I couldn't imagine my overweight mother doing the same. I made a decision at that time to grow old like my neighbor and not like my mom.

Unfortunately, many people learn the error of their ways only after illness has set in and they are forced to take a long, hard look at what time and the environment has wrought. Raphael Cabrera, described later, is one such American.

The medical and food industries try to convince us that we don't have the time or the taste buds for natural health. I aim to convince you otherwise. I am passionate about health and want you to consider your own health — or lack thereof — and discover noninvasive, pharmaceutical-free ways to lengthen and enhance the rest of your days.

Chapter 1: What Makes Us Sick?

From my associations with coworkers, friends, and patients, I've learned that when people become ill, whether it is diabetes, heart or lung disease, or even a common cold, they feel no responsibility for the illness that has stricken them. Either their genes are to blame or an infectious germ. And because they are ignorant about the causes of the maladies, they also are blind to effective cures by way of diet and lifestyle.

The Center for Disease Control (CDC) reports four risk factors relevant to at least 90 percent of all chronic disease: level of exercise, quality of diet, smoking, and alcohol consumption. Most people know that exercise and a well-balanced diet are good and that smoking and excessive alcohol consumption are bad. What may be a mystery is just what constitutes a balanced diet. We've been told for years to cut back on red meat and to eat a diet low in fat; hence all the highly processed low-fat food products that line our grocery store shelves. These recommendations are not based on science though and, in fact, may be significantly enhancing your chances of developing chronic illness.

In 1931, Dr. Otto H. Warburg received the Nobel Prize in Medicine for his discovery linking cancer cells to the presence of acidic conditions. If you know this (and now you do), all you have to do to ward off cancer and a host of other chronic conditions linked to acidity and inflammation is prevent acidic conditions from occurring within your body.

Everything we think and do contributes to the continuous acid-base balancing act that is going on inside us. In general, exercise (any type), raw vegetables, clean water, and meditation all promote alkalinity. Things that make our bodies more acidic include meat, sugar, grains, dairy, negative emotions, and immobility.

If this was known back in 1931, why still the ongoing effort to find the cause of cancer? This is what I've been asking myself since I started my own journey to prevent colon cancer, the so-called "hereditary" illness that runs in my family. I've even asked a few doctors this question, and the answer that I keep getting is, "people don't want to change."

What people want is not for the medical community to ponder. When it comes to sickness, it must be assumed that people want to get better and that they want to do it in the most efficient, safest manner possible. Medicine, if it's to be useful at stopping the occurrence and spread of human disease and suffering, must be based on science not shareholders. If science is demonstrating over and over again that diet and exercise are the best ways to assure a long, healthy life, the medical community needs to determine the most effective ways to get that message across. Rather than just push drugs while claiming it's what people want, the medical community should convince people to adopt healthier lifestyles.

I am certain the patients I care for in the ICU don't want to be to be poked and prodded by strangers 24 hours a day, nor do they want the dozens of medications with their numerous adverse side-effects prescribed to them. If people knew for certain their countless years of dietary habits adopted out of pure chance (or food industry propaganda) were what caused them to lie helpless in a hospital bed, and if they had the opportunity to replace those years of mindless consumption with better food choices and methods of cooking that would enable them to be healthy and vital, they would.

Research is continually demonstrating that lifestyle and diet are nearly 100 percent responsible for almost all chronic ailments. Yet food research is ignored by the conventional medical establishment, including the medical insurance industry that pays big bucks to treat diet- and lifestyle-induced illness without giving much thought (or money) to our diet and lifestyles.

Usually it takes about 30 years for new information to be accepted by the majority and put into practice. Information linking nutrition and exercise to good health has been around a great deal longer, yet excellent health remains an enigma decipherable only by a lucky few.

When is western medicine going to get on board and promote food as the pathway to better health? If poor diet and lifestyles are to blame for illness, it doesn't take a genius to understand that correcting diet and lifestyle issues will be the most effective treatment. Even better, these are the cheapest and safest treatments.

Having spent nearly half my life working in the thick of our healthcare system, it is apparent that our pharmaceutical-driven medical regime is reaping great rewards from poor health. The high profits are "just what the doctor ordered" for the highest grossing industry in the world. History tells us that diet and lifestyle are the culprits of chronic disease, and today's processed foods, along with our "pill for every ill" approach to health care, are contributing to early disease, disability, and pharmaceutical dependence.

Hippocrates (c. 460 to c. 370 BC) is considered the father of modern medicine. He refused to accept disease as spontaneous and out of our control and taught that illness is the result of environment, especially poor diet and lack of exercise. His words of wisdom have never been more relevant: "Let food be thy medicine and medicine be thy food."

In the early 1900s, after 100 years of being an accepted medical diagnosis, hypoadrenia (or hypoadrenalism) was removed from the medical establishment's list of accepted diagnosis, along with its only cure, diet and exercise (Adrenal Fatigue, James A. Wilson). The adrenal glands, walnut-size cones on top of each kidney, are responsible for producing hormones and stimulating other body parts to produce hormones that help us handle stress. Adrenal fatigue occurs when the adrenal glands do not function optimally. When this happens, the body is not up to the challenge of incoming emotional and physical stress and symptoms of illness begin to develop. These symptoms vary from individual to individual, but commonly include symptoms of thyroid disease, peptic ulcer disease, autoimmune syndromes, chronic pain and fatigue, as well as low blood sugar, a common prelude to diabetes.

Why did the medical profession choose to ignore adrenal fatigue and the health-saving preventative measures that are applicable to virtually every illness? Maybe because hypoadrenia is the precursor of nearly all illness and disease, and its only treatment, diet and exercise, is also the most effective treatment for nearly all illness and disease. If people actually recognized when they had hypoadrenia and treated it early with diet and exercise — the cheapest, simplest, and most effective measures available — we would have virtually no need for pharmaceuticals or long-term treatment for "chronic" illnesses.

Today's health treatment options (the ones that our health insurance plans pay for) treat disease as if the diagnosis itself is the cause of the problem. In other words, physicians tell you that diabetes has caused your unfortunate state of health and dole out diabetes medications that don't fix your causal problem but instead just string it along until other ailments arise. Diagnoses, once you start getting them, have a tendency to multiply, as do prescriptions.

If you have diabetes, I'm telling you that sedentary lifestyle and highly processed contemporary foods caused it.

If you believe your physician, you will dutifully swallow down your prescribed medicine with a diet soda at your favorite chain restaurant and then five years later wonder why your glucose-lowering medications have been increased or switched to injectable insulin, why you are losing your eyesight, and why your doctor is talking to you about kidney dialysis.

If you believe me, you will go to the gym and then stop at the local farmers market to buy fresh produce on the way home. Make this your regular routine, and you may never have to choose between hemo or peritoneal dialysis. This may seem profoundly different from what you're used to, but I think you will agree, daily green salads and 30 minutes of exercise several times a week beats regular visits to a dialysis clinic or frequent rounds of chemo.

Prior to the disappearance of hypoadrenia in the early 20th century, The Pure Food and Drug Law of 1906 went missing. Harvey W. Wiley, chief of the Department of Agriculture's Bureau of Chemistry, was a crusader for protecting the American food supply and the law's most vocal supporter. He believed the increased use of sugar and chemicals in processed foods was negatively impacting the health of the U.S. population. The incidence of diabetes and hypoglycemia (low blood sugar, a condition that frequently precedes diabetes and is also a sign of adrenal fatigue) were increasing at alarming rates, as was the amount of sugar and chemically laden processed foods Americans ate.

With the help of his "poison squad," a team of young, healthy adult males who were fed the same chemicals that were being used in processed foods, Wiley documented symptoms acquired after ingestion of the chemicals. He broadcast his findings on national radio. Unfortunately The Pure Food and Drug Law of 1906 so painstakingly supported by Wiley was dismissed when the Coca-Cola Company won subsequent lawsuits assuring its continued right to profit selling beverages containing potentially "risky" toxic chemicals foreign to your body.

Wiley's entire department was dismissed and replaced by the Food and Drug Administration (FDA), which became responsible for regulating and ensuring the safety of foods and medicines. Manuscripts written by Wiley describing unethical ties between political and food industry leaders disappeared, and Wiley was charged with multiple counts of misconduct. Wiley spent the end of his years (and I presume his money) battling in the court system and was ultimately exonerated before his death in 1930 (William Dufty, Sugar Blues, 1975).

That's how the FDA came to be in charge of the chemically laden foods and medications you and your family consume.

The food that Wiley was so desperately trying to keep off our dinner plates is the same food that the U.S. government uses our tax dollars to keep cheap and affordable: bread, crackers, chips and soda, highly processed packaged foods made from sugar, wheat, corn, and soy, as well as a host of chemical food additives that are negatively impacting our health.

Corn, soy, and sugar are genetically engineered, meaning their DNA has been violated by the addition of one or more genes from, most often, another species entirely. These substances invaded our food supply more than 20 years ago without labels and without any long-term studies to prove their safety. Now there is a great deal of evidence strongly suggesting genetically modified organisms (GMOs) are not safe for us nor our livestock, which are fed GMOs almost exclusively.

In light of studies in France, Canada, Germany, and other countries, the safety of GMO foods is highly questionable. Seventeen countries around the world have laws either prohibiting their use or requiring mandatory labeling to inform consumers. The state of California attempted to pass a mandatory GMO labeling law in 2013. Proposition 37 was the first of its kind in the Unites States, and even though it didn't pass (its opponents spent $45 million making sure it didn't), California's initiative increased Americans' awareness of genetically engineered foods.

Now other states are attempting to pass their own GMO labeling laws and finding the powers that be are still willing to spend millions to keep us ignorant. For whatever reason, there is strong opposition to letting Americans know what they are eating. Common sense tells us we won't know whether or not GMO food is negatively impacting our health if we don't even know when we are eating it. Labeling it thus would aid in its determination of safety, obviously something that should have been done before it was put on the market for widespread consumption. The FDA does support "voluntary" labeling, but thus far, nobody has stepped up to the plate.

In addition to being the most acidifying and pro-inflammatory foods on the planet, not to mention being made with unlabeled GMO ingredients, processed foods are addictive. Food manufacturers expertly tinker with their products, making sure they have just the right amount of perfectly blended rich, sweet, and salty artificially flavored perfection — with the sole purpose of hooking you like a cocaine addict. I saw it on a 60 Minutes episode, industry warehouses filled with perfume-size bottles of flavors and the depths to which food producers will go to make genetically engineered (GE) corn, soy, and gluten-containing wheat taste good.

Many registered dietitians and physicians insist you can eat anything "in moderation." The problem with the "moderation" approach is as long as you eat these foods on a semi-regular, "moderate" basis, you will continue to want them. An attempt to refrain from them, as in going on a diet, feels like deprivation and consequently you fall off the wagon. That's the nature of addictive substances.

If you are consuming highly processed breads and cereals, cookies, crackers, cakes, and the like (and why wouldn't you, since not only are they the cheapest foods because of the government subsidizations, but they also form the base of the food pyramid taught to many of us in grade school), you are acidifying/poisoning your body. Not only is acidic blood more apt to induce cancer, but it can also lead to a host of other malicious conditions that involve inflammation and premature aging. It's most likely happening to you too, even if you haven't been diagnosed yet.

Once you are sickened by our industrial food system, you get knee deep in the hypocrisy of our medical system, which rarely questions your food or health habits but encourages an assortment of pills and procedures that are supposed to help. The problem is that you never return to your previous state of health, no matter how many pills you pop. In my experience, both professional and personal, once people get involved with prescription drugs and start having medical procedures, negative health conditions spin out of control.

In the July 2000 issue of JAMA, Barbara Starfield, a physician with an impeccable record at John Hopkins University, presented research demonstrating 225,000 Americans die every year as a direct result of western medicine, including deaths related to complications of surgery and pharmaceuticals, making western medicine the third-leading cause of death in the United States following heart disease and cancer. Unfortunately, Starfield died in 2011 from a bleed in her brain, most likely caused by the combination of Plavix and aspirin, two platelet inhibitors she was prescribed to prevent a heart attack.

Starfield's research was never refuted nor has there been any new focus on re-creating a healthier health care system. When the majority of us are ill, we still turn to pill-pushing, western-trained physicians to diagnose and treat. They are, after all, the medical professionals who are reimbursed by our health insurance plans. Unfortunately, doctors are trained well in pharmaceuticals not food. When physicians diagnose an illness or label a group of symptoms, medications are certain to be the selected treatment, no matter what the original cause.

When the body malfunctions and requires an adjustment, you can be sure the blip is not the result of the body being in short supply of whatever drug the doctor has prescribed. For every diagnosis though, that's what we get, a prescription for a pharmaceutical, sometimes several. Treatment may be intended to be brief, as in the case of an infection, but even a short run of antibiotics can have far-reaching effects. If you're diagnosed with a "chronic" ailment, medication therapy is usually a lifelong sentence.

It's not uncommon for an infection to lead to one illness after another (and concurrent illnesses) — think "adrenal fatigue" — and before you know it, you are deeply encircled in the strong arms of the medical system and saddled with a half-dozen diagnoses. These "chronic" conditions are the aces in the hole for the pharmaceutical industry, because now you are certain to be a lifelong customer.

You also have an ace in the hole: your body is not static. "Chronic" conditions need not be permanent. We can undo the damage by changing our behavior and very possibly curing whatever ails us. It's as simple as this four-step plan for happy, healthy living:

- Exercise (any type)
- Eat raw vegetables
- Drink clean water
- Meditate

This is what's missing from today's "pill for every ill" approach to health care: it doesn't consider the cause. If sickness is a result of diet and lifestyle — and it is — then wellness is within our grasp.

The body is very forgiving, if we make simple changes in our daily habits.

Sure we have been told to quit smoking, to loose weight and exercise, and to consume at least five servings of fruits and/or vegetables. I read it in magazines scattered about the doctor's office, in between the adds for pharmaceuticals and sugar-laden recipes. But how much of our healthcare dollars are spent involving patients in fitness activities or teaching them that eating less of all types of meat (not just beef) is healthier and that vitamin C can help reduce the effects of smoking, alcohol consumption, and environmental toxins? How many western-trained physicians suggest daily vegetable juicing to their patients and recommend consumption of organic versus conventionally farmed foods?

I have been told on numerous occasions that I shouldn't be discussing these things with my patients, that it is the responsibility of the registered dietitians (RDs) to teach the patients about diet. But the Registered Dietitians Association (RDA) is heavily funded by the food industry, and consequently, the nutrition education RDs deliver is slanted towards highly processed foods, the kinds we need to be eating less of.

For instance, RDs will tell you to read food labels and choose foods with less sodium. I'm suggesting that if you really want to make a radical improvement in your health status, choosing foods without labels is key. I'm talking about broccoli, carrots, kohlrabi, or whatever suits your fancy at the local farmers market. It's best to stay out of big chain supermarkets that specialize in overly processed packaged foods, most of which contain not only GMOs but also toxic artificial colors and flavors that are meant to overpower your satiety hormones. In other words, these foods propel you to eat nonstop. Obesity anyone?

Our bodies can only function exceptionally well if we feed them exceptionally well: quality in, quality out. I know you're thinking organic foods are expensive and only the wealthy can afford them, but if you consider the cost of sickness, including the disability and medical dependency that go along with it, it's apparent that you get what you pay for. Pay the farmer or pay the pharmacist.

Despite the amazing effects a daily routine of exercise and fresh vegetables can have on our bodies, our healthcare dollars are spent on drugs and surgery. In emergency situations, drugs and surgery are great. They can and do save lives. But "chronic" problems need "chronic" solutions to prevent and cure, not just indefinite disease "management" after it has stricken.

Obesity, a huge problem in the United States and the world and one that puts you at risk for a host of other problems, is increasing at an alarming rate. Gastric-bypass surgery, the cure d'jour for obesity, is not the answer. I know half a dozen people who have tried it, but every one of them has suffered in other ways — from hair loss to chronic pain — and then regained their weight besides. Not only is there a risk of death on the operating table, I have seen patients of gastric bypass surgery die several years after their procedure from complications of adhesions. Development of adhesions is a risk associated with nearly every type of surgery and can lead to severe complications necessitating further surgeries months and even years later.

Insulin, Glucophage, amputations, and kidney dialysis are not the answer to diabetes. Lipitor and coronary artery bypass surgery (CABG) should not be the first line of defense against coronary heart disease. Certainly they are what most western-trained physicians practice, and some people do have positive outcomes. I just think it's weird that costly medications with significant adverse side effects and extremely invasive and expensive procedures are prescribed while the less-expensive, safer, and more effective means of achieving health are ignored.

As a young teen, I saw a 60 Minutes episode describing a research study in which cardiovascular heart disease was reversed after six months of an intense lifestyle- and diet-changing program that included strict vegan diet, meditation, yoga, and aerobic exercise. The participants in the study were informed they needed coronary artery bypass surgery but were given the opportunity to be research subjects instead. All but one not only survived but also successfully reversed their coronary artery disease and avoided surgery. I remember thinking how great it was that this kind of research was being done and assumed it would lead to us all adopting healthier lifestyles.

I couldn't have been more wrong. The consumption of highly processed "fast" food has steadily increased as has the percentages of nearly all disease states. Conditions of obesity, heart disease, pulmonary disease, Parkinson's, cancer, auto-immune diseases, and mental illness (yes the foods we consume also affect our mental well being) are not only increasing in staggering numbers, but they are reeking havoc on people's lives at ever younger ages. Too many people are suffering from too many diseases and living lives chained to the medical establishment. Even if this doesn't describe you (yet), it does or will describe someone you love.

And who do you think is paying for this medical mayhem? You are, with your heath and your pocketbook. The money being raked in by the pharmaceutical and healthcare industries is decreasing our standard of living and widening the gap that separates the haves from the have-nots. We could spend a great deal less and live healthier if the healthcare industry spent more time and money preventing illness rather than treating it with drugs and surgery.

You don't need to wait for the healthcare industry to get its butt in gear. You have the power every day to transform your health.

It may take more than consuming five servings of fruits and vegetables a day to transform your health, but that's a good place to start. Regardless of what medical treatment is chosen for your diabetes, hypertension, dyslipidemia, or whatever else ails you, if diet and lifestyle issues are not addressed, health conditions will persist. In many cases, unless dramatic changes in diet and lifestyle are made, life becomes a spiraling downhill roller coaster of illness and disease. With the addition of drugs and/or surgery, this downward spiral often picks up speed.

My own reality check of the sickening truth about our healthcare system began when my weight, cholesterol, and blood pressure all increased despite my long-time personal belief that exercise was going to save me from the common maladies of old age. In my 20s, before children, my average weight was 120 pounds, and I didn't have to spend much time or effort keeping it there. But in my 30s, after the births of my two boys, even though I continued my usual exercise routines of jogging and biking, I had a difficult time keeping my weight near 130 pounds. If I wasn't actively paying attention to every morsel of food I consumed, it would creep up to 140 pounds. I didn't think too much of it at the time because most moms I knew didn't maintain their slim pre-pregnancy figures, and I believed my long-time commitment to exercise would keep me healthy.

In my early 40s, my blood pressure climbed from 100/60 to 120/80 and total cholesterol from the 150s to the 180s. Though both were well within the accepted "norms" at that time (recent tightening of accepted parameters now make persons with these values candidates for both a lipid-lowering agent— statin — and an antihypertensive or blood pressure–lowering agent), these numbers along with my increased body weight demonstrated to me that exercise wasn't enough. I needed to do more if I wanted to exist into my 70s and 80s without crippling disease.

I looked at the rising values as putting me a couple steps closer to colon cancer, the dreaded disfiguring and fatal disease that is prevalent in my family history, and its most common surgical intervention, the colostomy. A colostomy is a surgical incision in the colon that is connected to another surgical hole in the abdomen where a collection bag for excrement is attached. As a nurse, I didn't mind caring for other people's colostomies, but I wanted to do everything I could to prevent having one of my own.

Despite my physician's assertions that everything was fine, I wondered what was causing my numerical stats to rise. Thus began my personal journey to optimum health. I read book after book, old and new, and very similar information kept staring me in the face. Whether they were written by medical doctors, nutritionists, biologists, or lay people who underwent their own health transformations, the connecting theme in all of them was food. I learned food has the power to make you well if you choose wisely but can allow your body to become riddled with disease if you don't.

How could I have forgotten about the vegan diet that helped reverse atherosclerotic heart disease? Maybe because I had been a registered nurse working in critical care for more than 20 years caring for hundreds if not thousands of cardiovascular-diseased patients and not one of them had ever been encouraged to adopt a vegetarian or vegan diet by the medical staff or the RDs who I worked with.

I came to realize that my diet, which closely matched the food pyramid taught to me throughout school, was not doing my body any good. The food I was eating was laced with hormones, pesticides, and artificial colors and flavorings, and it was prepared with methods of cooking that rendered many nutrients useless. If I had continued eating the way I had been taught, there was a strong probability of acquiring not only colon cancer but also a host of other ailments that are routinely attributed to the "normal" aging process.

I was shocked by the abundance of information linking vegetables to good health. If I consumed more vegetables and continued a moderate amount of exercise, I stood a pretty good chance of going to the grave ambulatory, continent, and oriented times three with all my body parts intact. It was a deal I couldn't pass up. If it's that simple why doesn't everybody eat fruit and vegetables as opposed to McDonalds? Why doesn't the healthcare system that I have been a part of for more than 25 years spend more time teaching people to eat better and less time poking holes and pushing drugs?

The powers that be, including our government, healthcare, and pharmaceutical industries, do not go out of their way to make it known that increasing consumption of vegetables and decreasing consumption of all types of animal products, especially highly processed meats, is good for us. Quite the contrary, when one starts poking around and asking questions, terms like "alternative health freak" and "quack" get thrown around.

Though I had no plans of saving anyone's health but my own, I continued on my "alternative health freak" journey. It took nearly two years of learning about the consequences of excess animal protein before I realized my own addiction to food, especially meat and cheese. It became amazingly apparent that my desire for meat and cheese had nothing to do with hunger. Every one of my favorite foods — cheeseburgers, tacos, nachos, pizza — included a combination of the two. Also painfully obvious was the fact that I consumed way beyond fullness when I partook of these favorites.

Because I valued my health and didn't want an addiction that I knew would lead to obesity, hypertension, diabetes, heart disease, arthritis, and especially colon cancer — all the various ailments that my patients suffer from — I finally adopted a vegetarian diet bordering on vegan, and my excess weight melted off. The first two months I didn't loose an ounce but felt great and less bloated. During the third month, I lost 10 pounds.

At first I didn't know what to eat and started by looking up various vegetable recipes in the many cookbooks I already had on hand. Then I sought out vegetarian cookbooks. Soon I discovered food tastes good even without cheese and meat.

Improving your diet does not have to mean giving up the foods you love; it need not be all or nothing.

Cow's milk is meant to fatten up baby cows; human babies are usually weaned off breast milk the first year. Thus it is common sense that dairy products should not be the cornerstones of your diet unless you're an infant. That doesn't mean you can't occasionally enjoy them. Sometimes the deprivation of not allowing yourself a treat now and then is what throws you off a perfectly good diet and into excessive indulgence. Be mindful of ingredients, because industrialized, chemical-laden foods are difficult to consume "wisely" without desiring more.

I don't promote a strict vegan or any other type of diet for everybody. Every body is different, but if health is important to you, be mindful of what you put into your mouth. If dairy, meat, sugar, and highly processed foodstuffs are the main ingredients in your diet, you need to continue reading this book.

If there was something I could do to prevent spending the latter half of my life tied to the medical industry, with a continuous regimen of drugs and hole poking procedures, I was interested. The more I learned, the more I tweaked the things I regularly placed into my mouth. I not only learned about new things to eat but also about new ways to prepare food.

All three of my vital stats returned to their previous low norms, and I learned beyond a shadow of a doubt that the current western medical establishment is barking up the wrong tree. Genes only predispose us to ill-health conditions when we don't treat our bodies with tender loving care. Carrying a gene is not synonymous with getting a disease unless you live a lifestyle that "turns it on," and you can pretty much expect disease and disability as a fact of nature if you live a lifestyle that does.

Watching the age of my patients consistently decline over time with preventable illnesses is intolerable, and I can't sit by and pretend I don't see the pink elephant in the room.

The food many of us consume is not safe, and the illnesses that result from it are treated with unsafe, ineffective drugs.

Current food traditions lead to disease and disability — do not pass go, go directly to the doctor's office and then the hospital, where, if you are 65 years old or older, on Medicare, and have a long list of medical diagnosis and prescriptions deeming you at risk, you may be assigned a "health coach" to help manage your elongated list of pills and doctor appointments. This is a new trend to help ease the cost of our disastrous medical system.

Health coaches are not a bad idea, but the best time to be seeking help from a health coach (or from a few good books on health) is not when you're 65 and already have a long list of health problems. The best time is now.

You and only you have the power to alter your head-on collision with "chronic" illness. Do it.

Quite surprisingly, it's simpler than you think. If you tried in the past and can't seem to get a handle on your health or your health goals, it is worth seeking out a health coach. Not only your life but your quality of life depends on it.

One definition of insanity I've heard is to keep doing the same thing over and over again while expecting different results. This describes the U.S. healthcare system that I have been a part of for the last 25 years. Rather than provide healthcare consumers with realistic information about diet, lifestyle, and the tools required to reach attainable health goals, we just keep admitting extremely sick people to the hospital and ignore what got them there in the first place.

Health care is the largest gross national product (GNP) in the United States, and pharmaceuticals are largely responsible for the continued increase in GNP devoted to health care. Not surprising, the pharmaceutical industry is among the wealthiest in the world. By doling out pills for every illness known to humankind, the responsibility for wellness, not to mention the "know-how," has been taken away from the individual and given to an industry that is making a fortune off of our sickness.

According to the Centers for Disease Control and Prevention (CDC), the United States spent $234.1 billion on pharmaceuticals in 2008, a figure that doubled since 1999 and increased to $329.2 billion in 2011. In 1950, healthcare costs made up roughly five percent of the GNP; in 1990, it was up to 12 percent. Currently the figure is upwards of 18 percent with estimates of 20 percent by 2020.

Most of the patients admitted to the ICU are on multiple prescriptions and are never expected to heal from their "chronic" illness. Instead, the list of medical ailments we suffer from grows steadily as we age, as does our list of medications. Those of us over 60 take five separate prescriptions each, on average. If medications are doing any good, then taking them should provide increased energy and vitality. That's not something my patients are experiencing, nor do I see much of it when I look around. Instead, at supermarkets, amusement parks, movie theaters, banks, and shopping malls, I see overweight people barely hobbling along, sometimes riding in carts because they are no longer ambulatory. No excess of vitality there.

Many of my patients come from nursing homes and have much longer med lists — 10 to 20 different prescription medications is not unusual. These patients frequently suffer from severe dementia, are immobile, and have no control over their bowels or bladder. I wonder what all the prescriptions are supposed to be doing for these patients, and I can't help but think the drugs contributed to their demise. I know what they are doing for the pharmaceutical industry. Money is money, and it doesn't matter who takes their drugs, the more the merrier.

Those who are willing to change dietary and daily habits will find even small, consistent modifications have major health benefits that surprise their doctors. My best friend's husband, Scott, was proud of being the only one of his coworkers who hadn't been prescribed medications. That is until a couple of years ago when he was told at a routine doctor visit that not only was he overweight, which he knew, but he had high cholesterol and was hypertensive to the point that it could not be ignored. Scott refused the prescriptions his doctor insisted on and instead opted to make immediate dietary changes.

The doctor didn't believe Scott could make the changes necessary to effectively reduce his vital stats and gave him only two weeks, after which time the doctor wanted him back in the office to recheck his blood pressure. Scott immediately gave up his norm of fast food lunches in trade for his wife's home-prepared sack lunches and limited himself to two beers after work in the evenings. Scott lost a few pounds and to his doctor's surprise, reduced his blood pressure enough to allow another two weeks to go by. At the next checkup, Scott was no longer hypertensive, and his weight continued to drop.

In other words, he cured his hypertension in less than 30 days simply by giving up fast food lunches, which he had been eating Monday through Friday, week after week. Six months later, Scott had lost a total of 30 pounds and his cholesterol was no longer an issue. He is 55 years old today and remains the only one of his coworkers who doesn't take prescribed meds. And by the way, he is the only one who brown-bags it.

Like the guy who lost his keys and went looking for them in the lamplight because that's where he could see, our healthcare system is looking for health in all the wrong places. The lamp lit area where it misguidedly searches is costly and invasive; lucrative for those in the industry but dangerous, sometimes disastrous for those caught up in its glare.

Besides being expensive, this healthcare methodology is detrimental to our health. Symptoms of illness are warning signals that something within our body is malfunctioning or broken. Squelching the symptoms with medications that don't actually resolve the problem can only lead to further health problems because the original health condition was ignored and now the body has more work to do metabolizing and detoxifying the chemical toxin known as "medication."

Take the simple cold. The best thing we can do to get over it quickly is to provide the body what it needs to strengthen its immune system. In most cases, this is simply rest and nutritious foods and beverages. But in our busy lives, we have so many things to do and no time for rest or even for nutritious foods, so instead, we use over-the-counter cold remedies to mask the cold symptoms while we continue our busy schedules. If we're lucky, this just leads to a prolongation of the cold, but if we're not so lucky, we end up with bronchitis or pneumonia or much worse if the adrenals are already maxed out from excessive stress and/or years of unhealthy eating.

The pharmaceutical industry has us believing we don't have any control over our bodies and must come to them for drugs to keep us "healthy." Yet their drugs don't cure; the majority of prescription drugs are intended to be taken indefinitely year after year until death do you part. The older you get, the longer your list of chronic ailments and the more pills you have in your medical regimen. Forgetfulness, there is a pill for that. Incontinence, they have something for that too. Stiff muscles, rub some chemical ointment on them. Every ailment that you could possibly think of has a synthetic pharmaceutical remedy that only covers up symptoms for a time.

Luckily, if you pay closer attention to what you eat most days and add a little exercise to your daily routine, you won't need any pharmaceuticals. If and when you do, there are less expensive, 1000-year old remedies that are safer to use. Where is the doc prescribing weight loss by means of exercise and organic vegetables? There is no financial gain for Big Pharma with this kind of prescription, but there are huge gains for you, if you value your health.

Some doctors practice what is called "Functional Medicine." They are medical doctors in every sense of the word, but they help patients use the nutrients in foods to restore health instead of prescribing medications to cover up symptoms. Functional Medicine physicians actually attempt to get to the cause of an ailment and treat the cause. Usually it has to do with ridding the body of environmental toxins (detoxification) and supplying it with needed nutrients. I was a nurse for more than 20 years before I learned of this practical method of healing.

Interestingly, Kaiser Permanente, one of the largest healthcare providers in the United States and one whose advertisements are continually proclaiming the preventative nature of their health care, does not have any Functional Medicine doctors on staff. Neither does UCSD Medical Center, Sharp Health Care, Palomar Health Care, or Scripps Health. These are the largest health care institutions in San Diego, California, and none of them have even one Functional Medicine physician on staff. Nor are they likely to recommend one as part of your treatment. If you're interested in improving your health, and preexisting health conditions necessitate the involvement of a physician visit the website for the Institute for Functional Medicine (www.functionalmedicine.org) and search for a Functional Medicine physician near you.

Chapter 2: What's Food Got to Do with It?

Carbohydrates, fat, and protein are macronutrients that provide calories for energy and building materials that form the structure of our bodies. The best sources of these substances contain trace minerals, vitamins, and other ingredients known as micronutrients that aid in the thousands of functions our bodies are continuously performing every second of our lives. Though our diets have changed drastically in the last century, to function optimally, our bodies still require the same nutrients that were found in the diets of our ancestors. The more modern and processed and out of balance our diets get, the sicker we get.

Sugar

One major change involves sugar, a simple carbohydrate also known as a disaccharide. Americans become addicted to sugar early in life. As infants, we drink sweetened beverages from bottles and sippy cups. As toddlers, we are rewarded with cookies and candy for being "good." Throughout our entire lives, birthday parties and holiday celebrations are filled with scrumptious, tantalizing treats that are as charming to the eye as they are to the taste buds — at least for the few seconds they are in contact with the taste receptors that line our tongues. After that brief moment of pleasure, then what?

According to Dr. Robert Lustig, MD, professor of Pediatrics in the Division of Endocrinology, and the leading expert in childhood obesity at the University of California, San Francisco, School of Medicine, the abundance of sugar and high-fructose corn syrup (HFCS) we consume leads to the accumulation of fat in and around our livers and ultimately to chronic disease. Unlike complex carbohydrates, which break down into glucose and are able to be metabolized by every cell in the body, only the liver metabolizes the fructose that makes up sucrose and HFCS.

When consumed, sugar is transformed into fructose and glucose through a process called hydrolysis. If the liver is bombarded and overwhelmed by high amounts of fructose, it immediately turns the sugar to fat. This is how we end up with fatty livers, even those of us who don't consume large amounts of alcohol. It is well known that alcohol consumption produces an abnormal amount of fat around the liver, but the news about table sugar inducing fatty livers is only recently becoming common knowledge, despite attempts by scientists like W. H. Wiley and others to sound the alarm. Unfortunately, the power of major food industry players has kept sugar's detrimental affects on the body largely under raps.

Fatty livers result in insulin resistance or metabolic syndrome. Metabolic syndrome has been singled out as the main culprit in obesity, heart disease, diabetes, and cancer. It kind of makes one think twice about all the added sugars that are present in processed foods, especially those marketed to children like breakfast cereals, canned pasta meals, sweetened beverages, and lunch-size snack packs of jello and pudding. These are the foods our young are raised on and sadly, the foods that lead to sugar addictions and an assortment of health problems later on.

These sugar-laden foods so entrenched within our culture are major contributors to the slow poisoning we unknowingly experience every day. I can't stress enough that we are not all created equal — for some, this poisoning is not insidious. Although many food-related ailments develop over years into easily diagnosable chronic ailments, others lead to acute autoimmune issues that leave doctors scratching their heads. Very few western-trained physicians bother to ask about dietary habits, and why would they since they are not educated in nutrition in medical school.

There are a lot of critics to the sugar-as-a-toxin theory and many of them are in some way profiting from the sweet white powder that Lustig proclaims is much worse than "empty" calories. Most agree, however, that at some point, the consumption of sugar is toxic. The question is, how much?

Take a look at just how much we are consuming today compared to 300 years ago. According to the United States Department of Agriculture (USDA), we each consume close to 150 pounds of sugar every year, which is 20 times more than we did in 1700 when seven and one-half pounds per year was the average. This doesn't take into account the difference between "added" sugars and those occurring naturally in foods.

In 1700, nearly 100 percent of the sugar consumed was in the food it originated from — fruits and vegetables. The slower digestion of dietary sugar in this high-fiber form is less of a threat to homeostasis. "Added" sugars are those that are introduced to food — sugars that are not present in their natural whole-food product state. They are typically added to low-fiber foods, which get absorbed quickly, assaulting our liver and biochemistry.

When we consume and digest sugar, our blood-sugar levels spike, causing the pancreas to secrete insulin, the hormone that drives blood sugar into cells where it can be used for energy. The more sugar we consume, the more insulin our bodies secrete and the more likely we will become insulin resistant at some point. This drives up insulin levels even higher. Chronically elevated insulin levels cause higher triglyceride levels and blood pressure, lower levels of the good cholesterol (HDL), and further worsen insulin resistance — in other words, metabolic syndrome. If you have an enlarged waistline, over 40-inch circumference for men and over 35 inches for women, this is suggestive of metabolic syndrome.

To avoid obesity, the USDA guidelines recommend Americans reduce their "added" sugar consumption to no more than eight or nine teaspoons per day based on a 2000-calorie diet. This is less than what is present in one can of soda, which typically contains ten teaspoons of sugar. Giving up soda and other sweetened beverages is a big step towards reducing your sugar intake and improving your health.

Unfortunately, many who attempt healthier lifestyles by reducing sugar intake turn to artificial sweeteners. NutraSweet, otherwise known as aspartame, is an example of a very popular artificial sweetener used heavily in diet sodas. It also is the most complained-about food additive on the planet, accounting for 75 percent of all adverse food effects reported to the FDA. Aspartame and monosodium glutamate (MSG) are excitotoxins that literally excite or stimulate neural cells to death, according to Dr. Russell Blaylock, a professor of neurosurgery at the Medical University of Mississippi and author of Excitotoxins: The Taste That Kills. His book explains in detail the damage caused by the ingestion of aspartame and MSG.

Sweet Misery by Dr. Joseph Mercola describes the deleterious effects of another artificial sweetener, Splenda or sucralose. Low-calorie, artificial sweeteners like NutraSweet and Splenda are not without deleterious health consequences of their own and are poor alternatives if one is attempting to improve one's health by giving up sugar. What is known about these and other artificial sweeteners is so compelling it amazes me that the FDA continues to condone their use. It is even more upsetting that hospitals distribute these little pink and blue packages of poison on patient meal trays as if they are benign. In my experience, patients are provided these substances and diet sodas in unlimited quantities.

These damaging sugar substitutes are what many of us turn to with the goal of consuming less sugar. One toxic substance is exchanged for another despite research indicating artificial sweeteners may be fueling rather than fighting the obesity epidemic they were designed to halt (Obesity, volume 16, issue 8, pp 1894–1900, August 2008).

Water is your body's beverage of choice. By replacing your daily soda consumption with water and drinking several glasses between meals, you just may reduce your appetite. Thirst is often mistaken as hunger. If hunger or a sweet tooth remains after drinking water, eat whole fruit and you will be well on your way to reducing your sugar intake as well as reducing your risk of diabetes, heart disease, and cancer. If plain water is not to your liking (many find it disagreeable) and adding a squeeze of lemon or lime doesn't suit you, make a large pot of weak herbal tea in the morning and consume it throughout the day. Consistently weaken the tea over time and soon you will be drinking the water your body needs to thrive.

To those critics who insist Lustig's claims about the toxicity of sugar are exaggerated and that sugar's only crime is that it is "empty" calories, I say it is preferable to err on Lustig's side. I have spent half my life caring for patients with complications of heart disease, diabetes, and cancer, most of whom are obese. No momentary pleasure is worth the years of pain and suffering that "chronic" illness brings. The fact that added sugar consumption has dramatically increased in the last 20 years may be one reason for the steady decline in the ages of my patients.

Wheat and Gluten

While on the subject of carbohydrates, I must speak to the implications of bread and its most common ingredient, wheat. Wheat is the primary source of gluten. It seems everyone these days is going gluten-free and in my opinion, for good reason. Gluten is actually a protein, the primary protein in wheat. Our food industry giants have deemed it beneficial to add gluten to nearly every food item on our grocery store shelves. You may not recognize it on a food label because it has many aliases: vegetable protein hydrolyzed vegetable protein, starch, malt, malt flavorings, and vegetable gum to name just a few.

In his book Wheat Belly, William Davis describes the chemical structure of gluten as being similar to that of morphine, which may explain some of its addictive and sedating qualities. He also informs us that today's wheat plant consists of at least 50 percent gluten, unlike the wheat plant of yesteryear, which contained only ten percent. It has been hybridized to include the larger amount because manufacturers of processed foods desire the soft, spongy, and chewy qualities it adds to those foods.

It isn't doing your body any good though and has been blamed for numerous ailments from head to toe, including colitis, irritable bowel syndrome, constipation, diarrhea, flatulence, mouth ulcers, abdominal pain, anemia, ataxia, epilepsy, fatigue, depression, arthritis, autism, autoimmune disorders, ear infections, eczema, headaches, migraines, heartburn, irritability, neurological disorders, psychiatric disorders, hypoglycemia, diabetes, osteoporosis, thyroid disorders, sinus problems…the list goes on and on. The gluten-free diet is not just another fad diet. People are recognizing gluten is not just a problem for those diagnosed with celiac disease.

Celiac disease is an autoimmune disorder where the ingestion of gluten leads to damage in the small intestine.

It takes between seven to ten years of suffering from a multitude of symptoms before a diagnosis of celiac disease is made, and it is estimated that one percent of the population suffers from celiac disease, though most remain undiagnosed. Many more are gluten intolerant and don't know it. Those of Northern European ancestry are largely represented among both groups.

My husband, Bill, is Greek, and neither of us suspected him of being gluten intolerant. Recently, he went on a gluten-free diet for Lent. In the past, he has given up alcohol, wine, meat, and a number of other substances for the same occasion. When a 70 plus-year-old male friend of his gave up gluten after reading Grain Brain by David Perlmutter and felt more energetic and vibrant, it convinced Bill to give it a try. In past years, Bill has always remained on his fast for the entire 40-day duration, but when it came to bread, Bill admitted it was the hardest thing he had ever given up. He lasted only 30 days.

During his bread fast, I noted Bill to be more on task about completing projects around the house, and I swear his hearing improved. I didn't relate it to his abstinence from gluten though until he returned to eating bread. Then I immediately noticed my old husband was back, the absent-minded, hard-of-hearing one who loves to start projects but not complete them. Despite my recommendation that he give up gluten permanently, Bill has not complied. His son, Josiah, though, after witnessing his Dad's experience and trusting my assessment, has gone gluten-free.

Omega-3 Fatty Acids

Another major change to our diets that may be leading many of us down the path of "chronic" illness concerns the fats we are not getting enough of. Over the past two decades, the media has brought to our attention the benefits of omega-3 essential fatty acids, mostly in the name of cardiovascular health. The blessings of omega-3s reach far beyond cardiovascular health. The broad effects of omega-3s may be due to their conversion in the body to prostaglandins (PGs), hormone-like substances that regulate the function of every organ and cell in the body. Omega-3s, if you are lucky enough to consume them, also form the cell membranes of every cell in the body. If not, other fats may step in and do the job, though not as well. Cell membranes are extremely important for proper functioning of the cells, especially in the brain, and omega-3s help keep them fluid and flexible. Not surprising, omega-3 supplementation has been found to be successful in treating an assortment of modern-day ills (Andrew Stoll, The Omega-3 Connection, 2001).

You may be wondering why something so beneficial and necessary for our bodies is in short supply. The specific nutrients our bodies require evolved over thousands of years as a result of what was plentiful at the time. Historically, omega-3 essential fatty acids were abundant both on land and in the sea, easily accessible to our hunter-gatherer ancestors. Our environment and our diets have drastically changed, but not our need for omega-3s.

Those fortunate enough to live near large bodies of water and eat sufficient quantities of "wild" seafood, a primary source of omega-3s, have significantly less incidence of cardiovascular disease and less of the many forms of mental illness, including depression, bipolar disorder, and schizophrenia. Decreased occurrence of dementia among the elderly has been noted among those who consume a diet rich in seafood. Stoll even links lack of omega-3s to the jaw-dropping rise of attention deficit disorder (ADD) among our children. Omega-3 essential fatty acids have been found helpful in mitigating the symptoms of rheumatoid arthritis, Crohn's disease, asthma, and diabetes. All this and omega-3 supplementation has never been found to cause a single adverse side effect.

Omega-3 and omega-6 oils are both essential

fatty acids, meaning we require them in our diet because our bodies do not produce them. The omega-6 oils are pro-inflammatory and pro-blood clot formation (both important bodily functions), and we get plenty in our modern diets because they are present in common plant and animal sources. To balance out the pro-inflammatory omega-6s, we need to consume an equal amount of omega-3 oils, which play anti-inflammatory and anti-blood clotting roles within the body. Balance is key. Herein lies the problem. Americans and others consuming huge amounts of animal products and highly processed foods made with polyunsaturated oils are getting bombarded with omega-6s with drastically low intakes of omega-3s. Thus we are wrought with diseases of inflammation and excessive blood clotting.

Supplementation is necessary because unless you consume wild, cold-water fish (salmon, sardines, and mackerel, for example) at least twice a week (7 to 10 ounces per week) or are enriching your diet with the micro green algae that fish feed upon such as spirulina, chlorella, and blue-green algae, chances are pretty slim that you are getting enough omega-3 essential fatty acids to maintain optimum health. Though shorter, carbon-chain forms of omega-3s are found in some plant sources (flax seed, chia seed, pumpkin seed, and walnuts), Stoll purports that our brains perform best with the long-chain forms of omega-3s found exclusively in water habitats. I've read a great deal about the benefits of a number of specific nutrients, but omega-3s are the only ones I am convinced I must take as a supplement despite my varied whole foods primarily plant based diet.

Protein

Animal protein is the third of the macronutrients I want to discuss, because many of us are getting too much. The ongoing misconception is that our bodies require a great deal of protein — the more the better. This is false, and too much protein is damaging. Americans (I presume other populations as well) are suffering from overindulgence in animal protein. Several years ago, Collin Campbell lead the largest nutritional study ever conducted and later wrote the book The China Study describing his remarkable findings. His research indicated consuming higher than five percent of our daily calories from animal protein results in a multitude of modern day ailments, including heart disease and cancer. Campbell demonstrated that cancer could be turned on and off in mice simply by adjusting the amount of protein the mice were fed. Forks Over Knives is a movie documentary that also discusses Campbell's work. Sadly, like most nutritional research that warns of our sickening modern way of life, potentially life-saving information is given maybe a minute or two of consideration on network news and then never heard of again.

Depending on gender, size, and activity level, our bodies perform best on approximately 40 to 60 grams of protein a day. One hundred percent of this can easily be supplied from plant sources; it would take 19 cups of broccoli to fulfill this requirement or three cups of pinto beans or one and one-half eggs or 11 ounces of walnuts or one ten-ounce hamburger patty. Our daily protein requirement is actually quite low compared to what Americans typically consume. If we have two eggs for breakfast, we've already exceeded our protein requirement for the day.

Another misconception surrounding protein is where it comes from. Every vegetarian gets asked the same question, "where do you get your protein?" Yesterday, at a restaurant, I noted the menu indicated an additional charge for a "protein source" for salads. I knew that it actually meant a "meat source" but it was written as if the salad greens, nuts, and goat cheese were not sources of protein. When people ask where my protein comes from, my answer is always, "from the same place horses and cows get theirs, from plants." I assume everyone must have been brainwashed (as I was) into believing animal flesh and animal products are the only protein sources on the planet. In fact, the highest protein source on the planet comes from the microalgae spirulina, chlorella, and wild blue green algae.

~~~~~~~~~~

Because both animal-product and sugar metabolism produce an acidic environment within our bodies, those of us who indulge in large quantities of both (less than what you might think) are increasing our cancer risk with every bite. In addition, to maintain proper pH balance, our bodies leach calcium, a base, from our bones. Thus, consumption of these substances in typical "American-size" quantities is conducive to osteoporosis, a significant problem that leads to other problems described elsewhere in this book. In the next chapter, I describe in more detail some of the common "chronic" ailments we suffer from as a result of what we put into our mouths.

Chapter 3: Sickness Sucks

The Centers for Disease Control and Prevention (CDC) states that over one-half of all American deaths occur in hospitals. From my experience in critical care, I know that many of them are dying with tubes and catheters sticking out from head to toe. The medical industry has designed tubes for every orifice on our body and even for places that previously had no openings. This array of lines and tubes allow for administration of food, fluids, and medications and the draining of bodily fluids and excrement. Even breathing is accomplished mechanically using a tube inserted through the mouth or nostril and down the trachea to the lungs.

Often patients lie in bed for weeks and even months with these tubes and lines, unable to move let alone bathe or go to the bathroom. Nurses provide for every human need required to live — not live well, just live — while the body's organs are supported and doctors try to figure out what to do next. It's not a pretty sight, and it is devastating to both patients and their families. It certainly is not something we would choose for ourselves or those we love. Unknowingly though, we are choosing it when we fail to make health a priority.

I have often thought a reality television show documenting what goes on when you're hospitalized would be helpful in getting people to rethink how they nourish their bodies. My work as a critical care nurse has afforded me the opportunity to witness firsthand the archaic methods of what is currently known as "modern medicine," and I have come to the conclusion that there is entirely too much slicing and dicing. Our bodies are like water balloons with differing thicknesses of membranes holding the water or "life force" in. Some individuals can withstand deeper and more invasive pokes before their bodies succumb to the stress of holes being poked into their flesh; others much less.

These very un–Star Trek–like surgical incisions, venous punctures, and the multitude of invasive lines and tubes used by our traditional medical regime cause inflammatory responses, which are part of the healing process, and serve as portals of entry for invading organisms. You never know how much poking and cutting the body can withstand before it looses its ability to initiate a healing response or ward off harmful bacteria and viruses.

Family members are often surprised when their loved one does not do well in the hospital, despite doing well and living independently right up until the surgery or "simple procedure" that landed them in the hospital. It is not well understood by the general public or health professionals that we come with our own networks of biological processes hidden from view, and it is impossible to know who will meet the challenges of these invasions and who will not.

The medical industry takes these holes, pokes, and incisions for granted. They don't seem to understand the depth of harm poking holes entails. There are always risks, they claim, but when a patient survives surgery or whatever hole-poking procedure they have undergone, it is assumed that the risks are gone as well. The public is led to believe that after a procedure, if they survive, their condition is resolved or at least not worse, and they will resume life as good or better than before. This is all too often not the case.

As far as the "chronic" medical problems that cause people to be hospitalized — diabetes, heart disease, cancer, strokes, hypertension — there is a greater than 90 percent chance that they resulted from lack of exercise and poor diet. Their different labels and symptoms reflect the same disease: the disease of living injudiciously, also known as the disease of modern diet and lifestyle.

The following are descriptions of some common medical conditions that I encounter every day. I want you to understand why drinking water instead of soda and preparing more meals at home from scratch is important. Believe it or not, these two simple steps plus the addition of several 20-30 minutes walks every week can prevent these "chronic" conditions from happening to you and your family. Already diagnosed? You may cure yourself from a condition your doctor said wasn't curable. Or you may prevent the acquisition of additional medical conditions since each illness, without proper treatment (nutrients and detoxification), can lead to another, like the domino affect.

Included in this chapter are conditions that I deem of most concern because of their growing numbers and long-term consequences (obesity and diabetes), because they have been around so long that people take them for granted as normal aging (hypertension and arthritis), and because they are the leading killers (heart and lung disease, cancer, and strokes). I also discuss mental illness because of its growing numbers and western medicine's steadfast reluctance to consider diet modification in treatment. Autoimmune disorders, which affect people of all ages, often striking suddenly without warning and with crippling results, are discussed as well.

Obesity

Obesity is diagnosed if you weigh 20 percent above your ideal weight; morbid obesity is 40 percent above your ideal weight. Either diagnosis is far from the inconvenient extra pounds that two-thirds of Americans carry around. This in itself can be devastating, but according to the CDC, the obese population is at enhanced risk of diabetes, heart disease, cancer, strokes, hypertension, arthritis, depression, kidney stones, liver disease, and erectile dysfunction. I presume this is a very conservative list. I note the morbidly obese nurses I work with have joint problems requiring knee replacements starting in their 40s, and I am certain it is from the extra weight and added stress their joints have to bear. Because obesity contributes to so many other health conditions, its steadily growing numbers make it in my opinion, the number-one health concern in the United States.

But it's not just a growing concern in the United States, worldwide obesity numbers have doubled since 1980 when 11 percent of the adult population was obese. Today more than 60 percent of the world population is either overweight or obese; more than 300 million adults and more than 18 million children under the age of five are overweight. The World Health Organization (WHO) defines obesity as a body mass index (BMI) over 30 and "overweight" as a BMI over 25. BMI is calculated as weight in kilograms divided by height in meters.

Western medicine's answer to obesity is gastric bypass surgery or a growing number of other bariatric procedures designed to rid the body of excess weight. The stomach, like most of our tissues and organs, serves an important function. It prepares the foods we eat for nutrient absorption further down the gastrointestinal (GI) tract. If not adequately broken down in the stomach, nutrients will not be adequately absorbed in the duodenum. Thus these procedures often initiate a host of other health problems that prospective patients rarely hear about or are downplayed so that patients don't understand their significance.

To prevent complications from poor nutrient absorption, those who undergo bariatric procedures are prescribed several vitamins and minerals. Even so, chronic nutritional problems are still the root of many of the post procedure complications these patients suffer. As with any major surgery, there is potential for formation of adhesions and strictures months and even years later. I have witnessed patients die in the hospital several years after their initial bariatric procedure.

Failure to loose weight and regaining of weight after successful weight loss is a common problem among these patients. The reality TV show My 600-lb Life documents several cases of morbidly obese persons who have undergone these procedures, and I find it interesting that in every single episode that I watch, in the end, the subjects require a great deal of help changing their diet and lifestyle in order to reach their desired weight loss goals. If that kind of help had been provided right from the start, it would have eliminated the need for life-threatening surgery in the first place.

Before going to the extreme of surgical intervention, the most common method of attempting to loose weight is to go on a diet. There are two big problems with this strategy. The first is how to choose from the multitude of diets available. The second problem I encounter all too frequently is that even when diets are "successful" with weight reduction, people sooner or later go off the diet and return to their old pattern of eating — the food habits that made them fat in the first place.

In my opinion, if a diet is "successful," there is no reason to go off it. Of course, in order to be successful, not only must a diet lead to desired weight loss, it also must be affordable and satisfying enough to maintain indefinitely.

Many of today's diets are available as ready-made meals sent directly to your door. These foods are usually too costly to continue indefinitely beyond the weight-loss period, not to mention highly processed, which is exactly what we all need to be eating less of. Other diets may be too strict or devoid of favorite foods, thus making them unlikely to be continued long term due to feelings of deprivation. That's why I recommend the program promoted by the Institute of Integrative Nutrition: start by adding in water, exercise, and fruits and vegetables and slowly allow these new elements to crowd out some of the less desirable foods items and habits of our industrial modern world. These changes need to be progressive and permanent, not something to give up once weight loss is achieved. In my experience, getting started is the most difficult step, but once you do, you'll find you are "into" things that are good for you rather than the opposite.

Diabetes

Diabetes is chronic high blood sugar that reaps havoc on blood vasculature with potentially devastating health consequences, including blindness, kidney failure, and painful neuropathy, not to mention cardiovascular heart disease and strokes.

Diabetes used to be known as "child onset" (type I diabetes) and "adult onset" (type II diabetes) but because so many children are acquiring type II diabetes, this nomenclature is no longer used. No matter what the type, there is reason to be concerned, because just like obesity, the incidence of diabetes is increasing and it too increases your likelihood of acquiring many other illnesses (renal failure, blindness, cancer, cardiovascular disease, and strokes to name a few). According to the American Diabetes Association, more than 11 percent of Americans over the age of 20 are diabetic, and this number increases to more than 26 percent in the 65-and-over population. If you think this group doesn't include you, just give it some time.

According to the WHO, there are 347 million worldwide who are diagnosed with diabetes, and of these, 90 percent have type II diabetes. This type is amenable to dietary and lifestyle modifications such as 30 minutes of moderate exercise most days and a healthy diet. Despite its easy fix, there is a global pandemic of type II diabetes, and deaths related to it are projected to increase by more than 50 percent in the next ten years. The CDC expects most of these deaths will be from diabetic-related cardiovascular disease.

Newly diagnosed diabetic patients (and those yet undiagnosed) commonly present to the ICU due to complications of diabetic ketoacidosis (DKA) and hyperosmolar hyperglycemic nonketoacidosis (HHNK). Both involve decreasing levels of consciousness (coma) as their names imply, and both can be deadly if not treated.

Long-term diabetics come in for infections of their feet or legs often requiring partial or complete amputations of limbs. By this time, they have already experienced a decline in kidney function and many are on kidney dialysis, either hemodialysis or peritoneal, which is continued throughout their hospital stay.

Peritoneal dialysis can be managed at home through a catheter that protrudes through the abdominal wall (often resulting in infection). The abdominal catheter is used for the instillation of as much as 2.5 liters of hypertonic dialysate or "dwell" solution. The dwell sits in the abdominal cavity for a specified time using the hypertonic solution and peritoneal membrane of the peritoneal cavity to filter out unwanted waste products and excess fluids by the principle of diffusion. The peritoneal cavity is then drained of the dwell as well as extra fluid and waste products. This process is repeated up to six times a day to perform the job the patient's kidneys are unable to do.

Patients may do this every night while they sleep. It is considered "convenient" compared to traveling to a clinic several times a week for hemodialysis to have a machine perform the task that our kidneys normally provide 24/7 at no inconvenience at all.

Commonly prescribed oral antihyperglycemic medications include drugs that cause the body to make or absorb less glucose (metformin/ Glucophage) or to produce more insulin (sulfonylureas/Glimepiride and glyburide). These oral meds are used by type II diabetics, as is the injectable medication insulin when the oral agents no longer succeed at maintaining a normal blood level. Type I diabetics rely solely on insulin to keep blood sugar levels in check. Some diabetics require very large doses of insulin to reduce blood sugar to desired levels.

Considering that high insulin levels are being blamed for metabolic syndrome, which exists in conjunction with insulin resistance, diabetes medications may, in some cases, be part of the problem. Insulin and sulfonylureas have been found to increase the risk of pancreatic cancer (Reuter Health, Jan 21, 2012) and insulin promotes increased risk of cancer growth. The risks from both the disease and its treatment are worthy reasons to maintain a healthy diet free of added sugars and the associated blood-sugar spikes that promote insulin production. Exercise is also of great value, because working muscles do not require insulin to obtain the glucose needed for energy.

Lung Disease

In my earlier years as a bedside nurse, chronic obstructive pulmonary disease (COPD) exacerbation seemed to be the number-one diagnosis that I encountered (lately "chronic" disease is an equal-opportunity employer). COPD is a breathing impairment that interferes with the movement of air into or out of the lungs. Emphysema caused primarily by smoking is the most prevalent of these conditions, but asthma and bronchitis are also forms of COPD.

COPD affects approximately ten percent of the world population or 64,000,000 people, and it was responsible for three million deaths or five percent of all deaths in 2005. In the United States, it affects five million people — over six percent of adults — and is the third-leading cause of death, claiming nearly 135,000 American lives in 2010.

With emphysema, primarily exhalation is restricted. Anything that restricts exhalation of carbon dioxide is going to limit inhalation of oxygen as well. The pathology involves lung tissue inflammation as a result of repeated inhalation of noxious agents, primarily through smoking. It is incurable, but progression of the disease is halted when one quits smoking.

Both of my grandfathers smoked for most of their lives and both suffered from this suffocating condition. My mother's father lived next to an oxygen tank, first at home with us and then in a nursing home for the last 15 years of his life. My mother's stepfather was lucky enough to avoid the nursing home and the oxygen tank. He was mean though and had no tolerance for children. I didn't know it at the time but his facial expression was one of constant "air hunger." No wonder he seemed not to like us grandchildren. It's hard to like anything or anybody when you can't breathe.

Because smoking negatively impacts the entire body, many ICU patients with COPD have numerous medical diagnoses and become what we call "frequent flyers" because of their ongoing readmissions to the hospital. These patients start coming into the hospital in their 50s and their hospitalizations become more frequent the older they get.

In the ICU, COPD patients are usually on ventilators and are kept sedated for days, weeks, and even months until their lungs are capable of performing on their own. After two or three weeks on the ventilator, it is customary to have the endotracheal tube removed from the mouth or nose and to place a tracheostomy (TRACH) through the neck. It's easier to keep the mouth clean (a major source of infection), not to mention more comfortable for the patient if they are awake. In addition, their feeding tube is usually removed from the nose or mouth and placed directly through the abdominal wall (percutaneous gastric tube-PEG) into the stomach. This is how they remain for several more weeks, being turned every two hours to prevent bedsores. With the TRACH and PEG in place, they are usually eligible for downgrading to intermediate care unless cardiovascular issues are making them unstable.

Recently I cared for a 67-year-old female with exacerbation of COPD who was just admitted the day before. She had been released from another hospital 30 days prior and during that previous admission she had been hospitalized for two months, during which she had been on a ventilator for one month. In addition to her admission diagnosis, COPD exacerbation, she was diabetic with a below-knee amputation and had a colostomy as a result of a bowel obstruction. Like I said, smoking is detrimental to the whole body, not just the lungs.

This woman could easily live another 10 years with frequent hospitalizations and numerous more tests and procedures. She came into the hospital from home, where she is attended to by her husband as well as a paid caregiver who comes in eight hours a day. I expect that soon she will be placed in a nursing home. She represents a very common ICU admission. I can't imagine living like this, can you? Now is the time to think about it, because now is the time you can do something to prevent it.

Steroids are commonly prescribed to treat COPD during exacerbations of the illness as well as bronchodilators administered using handheld inhalers or nebulizers for ongoing treatment. The long-term side effects of systemic corticosteroids are well established and include adrenal suppression, diabetes, osteoporosis, skin changes, mood changes, fat redistribution, cataracts, hypertension, myopathy (muscular impairment), avascular necrosis (death of bone tissue due to a lack of blood supply), and secondary infections related to immune suppression. Inhaled bronchodilators generally stimulate the cardiac tissue and are associated with increased risk of cardiovascular events, myocardial infarction (MI), or strokes.

Cardiovascular Disease

Cardiovascular disease is the leading cause of death in the United States and the world. In the United States, it affects between six and seven percent of the population and is responsible for 600,000 deaths each year. Worldwide it claimed the lives of more than 17 million persons in 2008, a staggering 30 percent of all deaths. The WHO maintains that 80 percent of heart disease is related to the same behavioral risk factors the CDC claims is responsible for at least 90 percent of all chronic illness: unhealthy diet, physical inactivity, smoking, and the harmful use of alcohol.

The most common type of cardiovascular disease, coronary artery disease, claimed 380,000 American lives and 7.3 million lives worldwide in 2008. Coronary artery disease is the buildup of atherosclerotic plaque inside the arterial vessels that supply blood to the heart, resulting in restricted blood flow to the heart muscle (myocardium) and subsequently causing myocardial infarctions (MIs, which are commonly known as heart attacks). Infarction translates to cell death. Thus an MI is the occurrence of cardiac muscle cell death and results in a loss of functional muscle tissue, which may lead survivors to experience the other two most common types of heart disease: congestive heart failure (CHF) and cardiac arrhythmias (heart rhythm disturbances).

An MI is a medical emergency that can lead to death or significant disability if immediate intervention is not sought. Even if interventions (coronary artery bypass grafts/CABG or cardiac stints) are performed in time to save lives, depending on the amount of cardiac tissue involved, drastic reductions in activity tolerance may result, thus limiting physical activity. Retirement expectations like increased travel and time with grandchildren can be abruptly cut short once fatigue and shortness of breath set in. Cardiac procedures to restore blood flow to the cardiac muscle in an effort to prevent or minimize the extent of an infarction include coronary angioplasty with the placement of coronary stints and coronary artery bypass graft surgery (CABG).

The less invasive of the procedures, angioplasty with placement of cardiac stints, involves insertion of a catheter through the groin to the femoral artery. The catheter is threaded up the aorta and into the heart and then into the diseased coronary vessel. A tiny balloon is inflated in an effort to force open the coronary vessel walls (coronary angioplasty), widening the lumen of the vessel where a stint, which vaguely resembles a micro "slinky", is deployed. The stint is supposed to permanently prop open the vessel wall in hopes of restoring blood flow to the cardiac muscle.

Patients undergoing this procedure remain flat for the duration of the procedure and up to several hours after to prevent hemorrhage of the femoral artery at the catheter insertion site. They are placed on antiplatelet or blood-thinning medications to prevent blood clots from forming in the newly placed stint. Without the drugs, clot formation and a subsequent heart attack is likely. On the other hand, the drugs themselves are dangerous and predispose those who take them to hemorrhagic catastrophes.

When more than one diseased coronary vessel threatens blood supply to the heart or if the vessel involved is the main supplier of blood to the left ventricle of the heart, usually a CABG operation is chosen. This is a great deal more invasive than what was just described. It involves cutting the sternal chest wall open and splitting the sternum, the central breastbone that is connected to the anterior ribs, with a tool that resembles my husband's jig saw. Then little pieces of vein that have been carefully dissected and freed from one or both legs are grafted to the occluded coronary vessels, bypassing the occluded segments. The patient is placed on a heart-lung bypass machine to supply oxygen to the body's tissues while the heart is chilled and placed on hold to allow the surgical manipulation.

If you are unfortunate enough to be the patient, after the operation, you will be admitted to the cardiac care unit (CCU) with an endotracheal tube connected to a ventilator and a Swan-Ganz catheter in an internal jugular vein in your neck for ongoing hemodynamic monitoring and frequent assessment of cardiac output. A nasogastric tube will have been inserted in your stomach and protrude out your nose or mouth, hooked up to continuous suction for drainage of the stomach to prevent vomiting, which is always a concern with any surgery involving general anesthesia. A Foley catheter for urine will be visible hanging on your hospital bed. Family members are never well prepared for the site of the lines, tubes, and machines connected to their loved ones. It can be very dramatic.

The goal is for the endotracheal breathing tube to be removed (extubation) within 12 hours and for the patient to be out of bed within four hours after that. This is often not the case. Many complications can arise that prevent a timely extubation, including post-op bleeding, renal and or pulmonary problems, as well as neurological side effects from the anesthesia or lack of oxygen flow to the brain. Generally the older, more deteriorated, and unfit you are, the worse you do, meaning you can be hanging around the critical care unit (CCU) for quite some time.

My best friend's grandfather had a CABG operation, and he was never the same again. It was the beginning of his downward spiral of decline, and though he lived for several more years, in my friend's opinion, his poor quality of life was not worth the effort. It bears repeating: one's treatment outcome depends a great deal on one's prior overall health status.

For those prone to sudden cardiac arrhythmias (sustained rapid heart beats), placement of an automatic internal cardiac defibrillator (AICD) is in order. You have probably seen external cardiac defibrillators at airports or seem them "used" on TV. Victims are shocked with defibrillator paddles applied to their chest wall while an electrical current is delivered causing their entire bodies to jerk. An AICD performs the same task but from inside your chest. It is an implantable device that often is combined with a pacemaker and is capable of delivering an electrical shock when excessively rapid heart rhythms are detected. You can receive a life-sustaining shock anywhere: the grocery store, the golf course, even while playing with grandchildren.

Laws mandate specific drug treatments when you are admitted to a hospital with chest pain and diagnosed with MI. Unless contraindicated, your physician must prescribe aspirin, a beta-blocker, an ace inhibitor, and a statin, but no law mandates education regarding the benefits of a vegan diet, yoga, aerobic exercise, and meditation. Exercising and changing one's diet, though proven to be effective at reversing atherosclerotic heart disease (and most likely other atherosclerotic vessels besides those supplying blood flow to the heart), is not well supported by the medical establishment. My neighbor, Richard, told me his doctor used the term "long shot" when Richard informed him that he wanted to use good old diet and exercise to reduce his weight, blood pressure, and cholesterol following an MI. Richard was successful.

Another treatment not supported by the medical establishment but used for cardiovascular problems and vascular ailments in general since the 1950s is chelation therapy. It involves a series of intravenous infusions of a synthetic protein called EDTA (ethylenediaminetetraacetric acid) that is known for its ability to remove heavy metals. It is the recommended treatment for lead poisoning. Chelation practitioners found that their EDTA-treated patients reported improvement in a vast array of vascular-related conditions after the therapy (including chest pain related to angina) and thus its use grew. The American Medical Association (AMA) insists the dangers of the procedure exceed the benefits and claim between three and 30 people have died from it.

This is laughable considering literally tens of

thousands of people die every year from conventional medicine. Chelation therapy has treated more than 500,000 patients and reports an 80 percent success rate with virtually no undesired effects. Its opponents deny its success claiming the "placebo effect" may be the cause for patient improvements because there are no double-blind studies, studies in which neither the patients nor the practitioners know who is receiving the actual treatment. To my knowledge, there are no double-blind studies for CABG and PTCA procedures either, because it wouldn't be feasible. The American College of Advancement in Medicine (ACAM), which offers chelation therapy courses to physicians, has long been awaiting cooperation from the Food and Drug Administration (FDA) to fund and establish research protocols.

Regardless, nonsurgical chelation therapy with EDTA has been salvaging the vascular system (not just the coronary arteries) of many would-be surgical patients who opt out of conventional medical therapy (or are denied it because of the high surgical risk). In their 1992 book Forty Something Forever: A Consumer's Guide to Chelation Therapy and Other Heart-Savers, Harold and Arlene Brechner describe the requisite modesty exerted by professionals in this field so as not to cause too much applause or attention toward themselves or the miraculous benefits this procedure offers. They are concerned Big Pharma and the AMA may choose to wipe out their competition and shut them down for good. The book is full of stories about patients whose lives were transformed as a result of chelation treatment. I would give this treatment some serious thought before going under the knife for a vascular occlusion procedure and believe the Brechners' book should be required reading for anyone with vascular issues who is considering surgery.

Drugs used in the medical management of cardiovascular disease pose significant health risks. The regular use of aspirin, a platelet inhibitor that potentiates bleeding, can make simple falls or minor automobile collisions result in traumatic brain injuries. Hemorrhagic brain injuries are even more likely for those who take Coumadin, a significantly stronger platelet inhibitor frequently prescribed for those with chronic atrial fibrillation, an irregular heart rhythm putting one at risk for clot formation in the noncontracting (fibrillating) atria of the heart. The presence of blood clots can lead to strokes, hence the need for risky blood thinners.

Beta-blockers decrease heart rate and result in decreased blood pressure and cardiac oxygen demand. Adverse effects of beta-blockers, other than those that are related to their desired effects (excessive slowing of the heart rate and excessive lowering of blood pressure), include insomnia, impotence, and increased risk of developing type II diabetes.

Statins are drugs prescribed to lower cholesterol, and it seems that nearly everyone over 30 these days has a statin prescription. Three of four men I know who received prescriptions for them stopped taking them because of the neuromuscular side effects. Muscle problems are the most widely known adverse reactions of statins. Others are memory and cognitive problems, pancreas or liver dysfunction, sexual dysfunction (seemingly every drug potentially causes this), and even cancer and diabetes. If these disadvantageous side effects of some of the most widely prescribed meds in the nation aren't enough to set you on a personal path to sustained health through diet and exercise, I don't know what is.

Strokes

Strokes, or cerebral vascular accidents (CVAs), are caused by the interruption of blood flow to the brain resulting in infarctions of brain tissue (brain tissue cell death). Commonly strokes result in the inability to move one or both sides of your body and the loss of speech or the inability to understand when someone is speaking to you. Strokes are devastating because they leave you disabled and dependent, unable to care for yourself. Frequently strokes cause the elderly (and not so elderly) to require chronic care in nursing homes. CVAs are strongly linked to the presence of cardiovascular disease and diabetes.

My grandmother, Bonnie (the one married to the mean old man who couldn't breathe), died at age 95, but she spent the last 10 years of her life in a nursing home unable to speak (aphasia) and with severely impaired mobility. Immobile and aphasic is a tragic way to spend nearly one ninth of your life, especially if you were an active chatterbox like Bonnie.

Globally, more than fifteen million people have CVAs each year, leaving more than six million dead and five million permanently disabled with loss of vision and/or speech, paralysis, and confusion. It is the second-leading cause of disability after dementia and the second-leading cause of death worldwide for those over the age of 60. For those between the ages of 15 and 59, it is the fifth-leading cause of death worldwide.

In the United States, CVA is the third-leading cause of death, killing approximately 700,000 every year, and it is the leading cause of disability, leaving 40 percent of survivors with significant disabilities requiring special care. Four million Americans are living with disabilities as a result of a stroke. In the Unites States, 28 percent of stroke victims are younger than 65; globally, 31 percent are younger than 65.

Bonnie had been a fairly active elderly adult with a significant sweet tooth. Her decline began after she fell into her bathtub while climbing in the bathroom window after accidentally locking herself out of the house. She broke her hip in the fall and spent some time in a nursing home after having it surgically repaired. Shortly after coming home from the nursing home, she had her stroke, after which she spent the rest of her life in a nursing home.

Her sweet tooth was significant to her decline. Sugar consumption results in decreased pH, or acidity, and to correct the acidity, calcium, a base, is leached from the skeletal framework causing osteoporosis. This is an especially common problem among the elderly in this country, especially females, who are affected nearly three times as much as males. Osteoporosis affects ten percent of American women age 50 and above (4.5 million) in the United States according to the CDC's 2005–2006 stats. But it's not just sweets causing the problem; everything that contributes to excess acidity in the body has the potential to weaken our skeletal framework by promoting osteoporosis.

It is well known that CVAs lead to hip fractures resulting from falls related to impaired mobility and balance. Less commonly known is that hip fractures increase the chances of having a CVA, which is possibly related to blood clot formation as a result of immobility.

Sugar wreaks havoc on a number of systems in the body and only recently has it been implicated in the direct development of atherosclerosis, which in turn increases risk for both heart disease and CVAs.

We all have to go sometime, but we need not end our lives as disabled and miserable as my grandmother, Bonnie. My eldest sister, Kristi, who cared for Bonnie as age and her dependency grew, told me she prayed to God not to take Bonnie when she first had her stroke. By the end though, Kristi was praying for God to take Bonnie. I know how she felt. It was extremely painful for me to visit Bonnie at the nursing home when I was in town. The slumped, nonverbal, decrepit lady who had once been a fiery agile woman of quick wit now drooled and frequently had tears in her eyes. It was very difficult to see my grandmother without feeling her misery.

Drugs to prevent strokes for those who carry higher-than-average risk include the platelet inhibitors described previously. Ironically though, as these agents help to prevent embolic strokes by preventing the formation of clots, they increase the risk of hemorrhagic strokes due to their blood thinning or anti-platelets function. It seems that you are damned if you do and damned if you don't. Either way, the industry of western disease care is raking in big bucks.

Hypertension

Hypertension is a type of heart disease that involves the entire circulatory system and involves excessive pressure in the arterial system. Like the water pressure within your pipes at home, this high pressure causes damage to the vessels that contain it and may lead to heart attack, stroke, aneurysms, and dissections of major vessels. Aneurysms are ballooning or bulging out of weakened blood vessel walls, which are at risk for bursting, causing hemorrhage and death. Even if you survive the hemorrhage, you may be left disabled from a hypoxic event caused from the interruption of blood flow to a major organ, the spine, or a limb.

Worldwide, hypertension affects approximately 40 percent of those over the age of 25 and was responsible for 7.5 million deaths in 2008 or 12.8 percent of all deaths. In the United States, hypertension affects just shy of 30 percent of the population over the age of 18 and 32 percent of those ages 40 to 59. It was responsible for 26,634 U.S. deaths in 2010, the 13th-leading cause of death in the United States.

The two numerical values in blood pressure are the systolic pressure (top number), which represents the pressure in your arteries when your heart contracts, and the diastolic pressure (bottom number), the pressure in your arteries when the heart relaxes. During the relaxation phase, the heart's ventricular chambers refill with blood.

When I was in nursing school, high blood pressure was diagnosed when the systolic pressure exceeded 139 or the diastolic pressure exceeded 89 on three separate occasions. As with cholesterol numbers though, the parameters have been tightened and now hypertension is sometimes treated with blood pressure exceeding 120 over 80.

Hypertension is called the silent killer because it generally lacks symptoms. Its claim to infamy is related to the secondary damage it causes when left untreated. Overwhelmingly, hypertension exerts most of its damage on the heart, resulting in atherosclerosis and coronary heart disease, congestive heart failure, heart rhythm disturbances, and cardiomyopathy (enlarged, stiffened heart). It can lead to these even in the absence of a myocardial infarction (MI) because the heart is forced to pump against elevated pressure. Hypertension also greatly increases your likelihood of having a stroke and may negatively impact all the body's organs because of the damage to arteriole walls that affect blood flow to all organs and tissues. For instance kidney dysfunction may occur related to damage of kidney vasculature.

It seems everyone these days has high blood

pressure. Hypertension is something I used to think was solely prevalent among the elderly, but now I am noticing it more among those much younger, even 30- and 40-year-olds. Several of my much younger coworkers take anti-hypertensive drugs, and I can't help but note what they are having for lunch: french fries and cheeseburgers frequently followed up with pudding parfaits for dessert seem to be the norm. Remember the lesson of my best friend's husband, Scott, who cured his hypertension in 30 days simply by reducing consumption of these types of foods?

Anti-hypertensive drugs include diuretics, calcium channel blockers, beta-blockers, and ace inhibitors. Erectile dysfunction is a common side effect of nearly all of these blood-pressure lowering agents. Weakness, fatigue, confusion, and depression are also common to many of them. Frequent cough is specific to the ace-inhibitors and can be severe enough to necessitate stopping the drug for many people. In many cases, the treatment may seem worse than the disease.

Cancer

Cancer is the third-leading cause of death in the United States, killing nearly 600,000 Americans in 2014. More than 13 million Americans carry a diagnosis of cancer, of which only 66 percent survive five years. In 2012, cancer led to 8.2

million deaths worldwide, and like many other ailments of our time, the numbers are expected to continue to increase. The American Cancer Society reports a one-in-two chance of developing cancer for men and a one-in-three chance for women.

Cancer is unregulated cell growth leading to tumors, which may spread to other parts of the body (malignant tumors) and interfere with bodily functions. You are probably aware of the devastating consequences a diagnosis of cancer brings. Treatments are not only disfiguring but often deadly. I've already mentioned my own health research began as an attempt to prevent colon cancer, the health hazard most prevalent in my own family history.

The most common types of cancer reported in the United States and globally are lung, liver, stomach, colorectal, prostate, and breast. In addition to radically diverting the pathway of excrement after a colectomy (surgical removal of part or the entire colon), cancer causes one in four Americans to undergo mastectomies (removal of one or both breasts), hysterectomies (uterus removal), oophorectomies (removal of one or both ovaries), prostatectomies (removal of the prostate), lobectomies or pneumonectomies (removal of a lung lobe or an entire lung respectively), nephrectomies (kidney removal), and esophagectomies (removal of the esophagus). In this latter procedure, either the stomach is displaced up to the neck region or a section of colon is translocated to the esophagus region.

Sound like anything you'd want? I didn't think so. Then eat your vegetables, drink water not soda, and go for walks daily. It's a small price to pay to maintain your body parts.

Chemotherapy (chemo) is deadly. That's how it works against cancerous growths — it kills them. The problem is that its deadly toxins are not selective and sometimes you die in the process, too. If you do survive, the effects of chemo can make you so sick that you may wish you were dead.

I recently met Fred, a 69-year-old man who two years ago was told he had prostate cancer. His prostate-specific antigen (PSA) level was noted to be 4.2 after a routine physical. PSA is a protein produced by the prostate. Elevated levels (greater than 4) may be indicative of prostate cancer. Subsequent biopsy found Fred to have what he was told was a "very aggressive" form of prostate cancer, and he was operated on within one week of his initial doctor visit.

Prior to the operation, he was told of a myriad of potential problems that could occur with the surgery, but they were presented as "rare" complications. Today Fred is impotent with significant urinary incontinence as a result of the surgery and radiation. He is angry. The reaction he gets from his doctors is that he should be happy to be alive. But this man tells me he would have preferred to "live it up" for six months and let nature take its course rather than live with these troublesome complications. In my experience, the misfortunate outcome that Fred is experiencing is not rare at all, but actually a common result of prostate surgery.

The presence of cancer cells is a normal part of being alive. They only become problematic when our immune system fails to recognize and eliminate them. As we age, our cellular-repair mechanisms work less effectively, but that doesn't mean we have to just sit by and hope for the best. Though we can't stop the years from passing us by, we can pay close attention to the five leading behavior and dietary risk factors for cancer as reported by the WHO:

1. Increased BMI
2. Low fruit and vegetable consumption
3. Lack of physical exercise
4. Tobacco use
5. Alcohol use

Remember Otto Warburg and his Nobel Prize discovery linking cancer cells to acidic conditions (See Chapter 1)? If getting into your skinny jeans isn't enough motivation to loose the fat, maybe understanding that your excess fat may cause you to loose your breasts or some other part of your body. It is much easier to avoid cancer than to cure it.

Arthritis

Arthritis is another condition that I used to believe only happened to the elderly, but like hypertension, I'm seeing and hearing of much younger people becoming afflicted. The word arthritis means joint inflammation. The CDC uses the term arthritis in the public health world to describe more than 100 rheumatic diseases and conditions that affect joints, the tissues that surround the joints, and other connective tissue. The pattern, severity, and location of symptoms can vary, depending on the specific form of the disease. Typically, rheumatic conditions are characterized by pain and stiffness in and around one or more joints. The symptoms can develop gradually or suddenly. Due to the severity of symptoms, arthritis is a leading cause of disability in the United States and the world.

According to the CDC, one in five or 22.7 percent of the U.S. adult population suffers from some form of arthritis (2010–2012 stats), a total of nearly 50 million people. One in four will develop hip arthritis, two-thirds of the obese population will develop knee arthritis, and nearly one-half of people 65 and older (49.7 percent) will suffer from some form of arthritis. Peak age of onset is between 30 and 55. Globally, arthritis affects approximately one percent of the world population, hitting developing world populations hardest. In the United States and globally, women are generally twice as likely to suffer from it as men.

Treatment of arthritis is primarily with pharmaceuticals to manage pain and inflammation. Nonsteroidal anti-inflammatory drugs to ameliorate arthritic pain are rot with negative side effects like kidney failure and bleeding gastric ulcers. Narcotics are habit forming, tend to cause chronic constipation, and do not treat the inflammation. Chronic use of Tylenol is known to be toxic to the liver.

Even the CDC understands the influence of diet and lifestyle in the development of arthritis and recommends prevention strategies by reducing intake of sugar, increasing consumption of vegetables, and engaging in regular exercise. In other words, the same types of things that prevent cancer, heart disease, and strokes help to prevent arthritis. How convenient.

Mental Illness

The CDC defines mental illness as "all diagnosable mental disorders or health conditions that are characterized by alterations in thinking, mood or behavior or some combination thereof, associated with distress and/or impaired functioning." Depression is the most common type of mental illness in the

United States and the world, affecting 26 percent of the U.S. adult population and just over four percent of the global population. The diagnosis of depression is steadily increasing, and it is projected that by the year 2020, depression will be the second-leading cause of disability through out the world, second only to heart disease.

The CDC also reports that development of mental disorders, especially depressive disorders, are strongly related to many "chronic" diseases, including diabetes, cancer, cardiovascular disease, asthma, and obesity, as well as risk behaviors for "chronic" disease such as physical inactivity. Furthermore, the risk of death from all causes is increased in the depressed person. Depressed persons are two times more likely to die prematurely from any cause and four times more likely to experience a heart attack than the general population.

Our healthcare system prescribes a host of medications for numerous types of mental illness, and just like the drugs prescribed for physical health problems, mental health prescription drugs do not cure the problem. When these drugs are successful, symptoms are usually alleviated only temporarily. Typically, medications and their dosages require frequent adjustment and still are not successful or offer only partial relief of symptoms.

Like many drugs, those prescribed for mental

illness are extremely harsh to the body's organs, which may explain why I see so many mentally ill patients in the critical care unit with organ dysfunction in their 40s and 50s. Every one of them has a long list of physical ailments they've managed to acquire in their relatively short life. It's extremely disheartening to care for these patients, as I know the drugs they were told would relieve their symptoms may have made it easier for their caregivers but did not necessarily offer much help for their acute mental illness.

Our medical establishment does not consider poor nutrition as a potential cause of mental illness despite the fact that numerous nutrient deficiencies are known to cause the symptomology that the mentally ill suffer from. For example, according to Wikipedia, signs and symptoms of scurvy (vitamin C deficiency) include fatigue, exhaustion, depression, anxiety, and irritability. Likewise a biotin deficiency is a lack of vitamin B7 and can cause hallucinations and depression. Low B12 levels cause fatigue, irritability, and depression and can lead to more significant mental disorders if not treated. Lack of L-tryptophan, an essential amino acid, causes depression in just five days.

Iodine, selenium, and magnesium deficiencies may cause signs and symptoms of hypothyroidism, which include fatigue, depression, and constipation. Altered bowel habits often coincide with mental disturbances;

in the alternative health community, the gut is considered the "second brain."

The Washington Post recently reported the link between our gut and our brain and attributes the connection to gut bacteria ("Can What You eat Affect Your Mental Health?" March 24, 2014). The article begins with the description of a long-time sufferer of depression who had been on anti-depressants for several years. In an attempt to loose weight, the subject significantly altered her diet by increasing consumption of fresh fruits and vegetables. In addition to weight loss, she experienced a dramatic improvement in her mental status and successfully weaned off anti-depressants. The article goes on to say that more research is needed to determine if less-processed foods can improve our mental health. Yes, more research is great, but you may be waiting a very long time in a sorrowful state of health if you're planning to wait until all the data is in.

Dr. Andrew Stoll describes the successful use of omega-3 supplementation for managing several conditions of mental illness in his 2001 book, The Omega-3 Connection, and convincingly describes why this nutrient, severely lacking in the diets of the developed world, may be the hidden key to many illnesses. Its role in the prevention of heart disease is recognized by many, and in light of the close connection between heart disease and depression, it's understandable that omega-3s could be valuable in treating depression as well.

Dr. Stoll points out, as do many other physician authors of health books I've read, that pharmaceutical companies spend a great deal of money researching potential drugs that they stand to make significant profits from. On the other hand, naturally occurring compounds like vitamins and essential fats are not patentable and thus, for-profit industries are not likely to spend money researching their effectiveness.

Don't put your health on hold. You don't need to wait. There is no time more precious than the here and now, and fresh fruits and vegetables and omega-3 supplements are available now. Food is cheap, compared to pharmaceuticals, even organic unprocessed whole foods and high-quality omega-3–dense wild salmon or krill oils. Furthermore, these foods have no worrisome side effects. Eat well now and know that your body will benefit from head to toe, both physically and mentally.

Dr. Stoll wrote in his book that the medical profession is starting to recognize and acknowledge the benefits of correcting nutritional deficiencies when treating disease. Unfortunately his book was written more than 10 years ago, and I haven't noticed any monumental strides in the medical profession towards supporting food as medicine. In fact, I have had two disheartening conversations with psychiatrists about food potentially worsening my son's psychiatric problems.

The first conversation was about gluten. I pointed out to my son's psychiatrist that I read that gluten may contribute to mental instability and influence depression and schizophrenia. It has been studied since the 1950s when an unusually high prevalence of celiac disease was noted among hospitalized psychiatric patients. The psychiatrist did not look me in the eye when she told me she had never heard of such a thing nor would she even glance at the stack of research articles I brought to her office concerning the study of gluten and mental illness. The fact that my son's odd behavior was potentiated immediately following consumption of high-gluten meals and significantly improved by going gluten-free was not of any significance to her.

Another psychiatrist I tried to speak with concerning my son's constipation issues flat out said she did not treat that end of the body and was not interested in his bowel habits. Evidently she did not get the memo that the gut is the second brain and that anything that affects one will affect the other. My biggest criticism about western medicine is the asinine division of the body into compartmentalized organs with a separate physician to care for each one. It's as if the body and all its organs are not being supplied by the same blood, and the blood is not being supplied by the same nutrients. It's just another way the apothecary system dismisses the importance of nutrition.

Dementia

Dementia is an umbrella term for a group of cognitive disorders common to older adults, usually 60 years and older, typically involving memory impairment as well as marked difficulties in the area of language and motor activity. Dementia is the leading cause of dependency and disability among older people. According to the WHO, in 2010, there were 35.6 million people worldwide suffering these debilitating symptoms, with a new case occurring every four seconds. Between two and ten percent of persons living with dementia are younger than 65 years old. Physical, emotional, and economic pressures tend to overwhelm family members involved in their care, which generally include the surviving spouse or adult children.

Alzheimer's is the most common of the dementias. Alzheimer's disease (AD), per the CDC, is a progressive disease of the brain that begins with memory loss and eventually leads to decreased decision-making ability, inability to recognize loved ones, and inability to perform activities of daily living.

Starting at age 65, the risk of developing AD doubles every five years, and by age 85, between 25 and 50 percent of us will exhibit signs and symptoms of Alzheimer's disease. The CDC reports that currently 5.3 million in the United States are living with the difficulties of AD, and the number is expected to more than double by 2050 due to the aging of the population. Alzheimer's disease is the sixth-leading cause of death in the United States and is the fifth-leading cause of death among persons age 65 and older.

The CDC reports pharmaceuticals have not demonstrated success in forestalling the usual progression of dementia disorders, which appear to be related to the development of plaques in the brain. Chelation anyone? Chelation treatments were found to improve brain function of those suffering from dementia, but you're not likely to hear about it from your doctor.

Despite lack of positive results, doctors prescribe a number of drugs to cognitively impaired elder adults in hopes of slowing progression of their illness. The drug I see most commonly prescribed for patients with dementia or memory loss is Aricept (donepezil), a cholinesterase inhibitor. Its most common side effects are nausea, vomiting, diarrhea, weight loss, and insomnia. Elderly persons already tend to have trouble eating sufficiently (possibly related to decreased sense of smell or problems with chewing) and they also tend to have trouble sleeping. Thus treatment with Aricept may not be worth these side effects, especially if no improvement in memory is recognized.

According to the CDC, the same preventative behaviors that reduce the risk of heart disease, stroke, diabetes, and arthritis (increased physical activity and a diet rich in fruits and veggies) may also lessen the risk of AD. Omega-3 essential fatty acids may be helpful as well, according to Dr. Andrew Stoll, and with no deleterious side effects. Are you convinced yet?

The development of dementia among the aging population and the frequent need for home assistance or placement of the elderly in skilled nursing facilities is how retirement savings are frequently spent. This is because Medicare and Medicaid insurance programs do not pick up these expenses until one's personal funds have been exhausted. We are dying sick, depressed, disabled, and broke. But it's not written in stone; there are steps you can take to help prevent these hazards. Contrary to popular belief, they need not be part of the "normal" aging process.

Autoimmune Disorders

The CDC reports the existence of more than 80 autoimmune conditions. They are the leading cause of death for women under the age of 65. An autoimmune condition is one in which healthy tissue is damaged or destroyed by the body's own immune system, the system which under normal conditions selectively destroys bacteria, viruses, or other foreign proteins.

The tissues damaged in autoimmune disorders typically involve blood vessels, connective tissues, endocrine glands, joints, muscles, red blood cells, and skin; signs and symptoms vary. Two of the most common forms of autoimmune disorders are type I or child-onset diabetes and rheumatoid arthritis. Drugs prescribed for autoimmune diseases involve weakening the overactive immune system. This can have deleterious side effects, including the most obvious, a weak immune system that is unable to combat bacterial, viral, and fungal infections nor destroy ever-present irregular cells that consequently may develop into cancer.

Dr. Andrew Stoll describes the role an essential fatty acid imbalance between omega-3 and omega-6 oils plays in the development of chronic disease, including those that are considered to be autoimmune.

The Standard American Diet (SAD) of fried and highly processed ready-made foods is overabundant in omega-6 oils and significantly lacking in omega-3s. Both are essential, but balance is key. Consumption of omega-3 oils should equal omega-6 oil consumption one to one, according to Stoll. When we consume whole plant foods undistorted by the manipulation of the food industry, as well as foods from water sources either as algae and seaweed or fish that make their diet from these, we naturally consume the correct balance of these essential nutrients. On the other hand, meat, dairy, and processed foods contain excessive amounts of the omega-6 variety, an essential fatty acid, yes, but one most of us devour in outrageous quantities in the absence of omega-3s.

~~~~~~~~~~~~~

In most cases of "chronic" illness, no matter what disease brings you to the hospital, even if you manage to go home, chances are you'll be back again and again before you die. First though, you will spend a great deal of money on medical expenses.

It is apparent that the sickness running rampant all around us, affecting the health and livelihood of ourselves as well as those we love, results from diets lacking nutrient-dense foods and sedentary lifestyles. Don't despair. You and only you have the power to choose a different path and significantly diminish your chances of developing the wide assortment of illnesses plaguing so many of us today. First you must recognize the need for a change, and once you do this, the possibilities in health transformation for you and your family can become a reality.

If you are serious about improving your chances of aging without the development of chronic disease, you need to throw out the processed foodstuffs and add some form of exercise to your daily routine. You know what's ahead if you don't.

The devastating and potentially terminal health conditions reviewed in this chapter can be prevented. The choice is yours. If you're not able to reach your health goals on your own, it might be worth investing in a health coach to help you get started. Your life and quality of life are at stake. The next chapter describes simple, no-brainer activities that anyone can do to live healthier.

Chapter 4: New Game Plan

Common-sense medicine, what I call "self-health" is widely available to everyone at a very low cost and has no adverse side effects. This is what should be driving our healthcare system instead of high-cost, invasive, and dangerous procedures and toxic, expensive pharmaceuticals. Instead, alternative health practitioners have been criticized for their adherence to the concept of healthy living.

Orthorexia is when "healthy" eating becomes excessive. The question is, who determines what is excessive? Occasionally, I was ribbed at work for my homemade, raw vegan meals (fresh-squeezed vegetable juices and a variety of salads), mostly by those who ate fried foods every day for lunch. From their perspective, my healthy eating habits must seem over the top compared to their own choices. On the other hand, seeing french fries or onion rings on their plates every day next to a juicy hamburger or sandwich filled with processed deli meats with a hefty portion of dessert on the side is appalling to someone like me who vividly sees the direct harm of each mouthful. I sit quietly by, minding my own business while my eyes take in the tragedy.

The jeering has stopped, and now the worst offenders actually come to me for advice. Too bad the advice they are looking for is the same as they seek from a pill-prescribing physician. What single food or herb is going to cure them of their ailment of the day, week, or lifetime? There is no silver bullet. The answer is oxygen (aerobic exercise, muscle strengthening, and stretching), water (clean, nonfluoridated), sun (unfiltered by chemical-laden sunblock that is directly absorbed into your blood and tissues through the skin, the body's largest organ), unprocessed organic plant food, and nurturing relationships. These are the basics of good health. There are no shortcuts.

If you are seriously ill and anxious to get back to a healthier you, you might be tempted to go for the quick fix. If you are not in a hurry, a slow stroll down save-your-body boulevard might be just the ticket to ensure you don't become my next critical care admission. Either way, the only thing you stand to loose is sickness, suffering, and premature death. It's never too late, and it's always worth your efforts.

Exercise

My own health-seeking behaviors span more than 40 years, starting with that first observation of my elderly, jogging neighbor. I first started jogging in seventh grade because I thought my thighs were too fat. Now I run and bike up mountains because it's fun and because it keeps me feeling and looking my best. If cycling or running isn't your style, try parking as far away as possible from your destination and walk the extra distance — consider it a healthy indulgence. With gas prices as high as they are, I assume everyone who can is using public transportation and walking the distances between stops. Aren't they? Quit using elevators today and take the stairs instead from now on. Believe it or not, these small additions to your daily routine can have huge payoffs. Every little bit helps. There's no need to train for a 10K race unless the camaraderie among fellow athletes is what lights you up and drives you to maintain fitness.

I've read that just five to ten minutes a day jumping on a mini-trampoline is especially good for increasing oxygen intake and enhancing drainage of the lymphatic system, an adjunct to the circulatory system that is involved with filtering and detoxification as well as transporting immunological cells. Jumping rope can accomplish the same benefit, as will any exercise that involves up-and-down rhythmic motion.

Alternatively, you may choose to spend some time every day playing with your children (or grandchildren) or tidying up the house or working on home improvement projects. Take a dance class or karate. There are endless ways to get your body moving towards a healthier and more active life. Do it, and do it regularly. The payoff is your health.

Water

I didn't discover the health enhancement of food and water until my 40s. Food seemed obvious, but I had no idea about the benefits of water until I met a gentleman at a local winery who claimed to have cured his father of colon cancer through diet and lifestyle. I faithfully listened as he recommended drinking a liter of distilled water first thing in the morning as the most important change one could make to prevent cancer.

So began my morning ritual, though I used bottled drinking water and later reverse-osmosis water rather than distilled water. This trick alone melted off five pounds, not only because of the calorie-free water, but because of the resultant increased frequency and volume of my bowel movements. Weight loss and improved bowel evacuation are wonderful additional benefits to drinking more water.

Since then I've learned of the alkalizing benefits of adding fresh-squeezed lemon juice to my water. Its natural vitamin C (not the kind synthesized in a laboratory) attaches to and helps remove toxins from the body. Vitamin C is one of the main ingredients in our bodies' built-in detoxification system. Thus two, three, or even four eight-ounce glasses of water first thing in the morning with one to two lemons squeezed into them does the body wonders. I call it my mini morning detox.

Now I too highly recommend drinking water first thing in the morning as well as throughout the day. It is one of the best things you can do for your body. In fact, if you do nothing more than exercise, drink plenty of water, and abstain from sugary and artificially sweetened beverages, I am certain you will notice a remarkable difference in your health. Your complexion and/or your allergies may clear up, you might loose some (or all) of the weight you have wanted to loose, certainly, you'll feel better. If you just switch from sugar drinks to water, you will note immediate improvement in your overall health. Our bodies are made of mostly water, and every biological process they perform is enhanced when they are well hydrated.

Raw Foods

The best water on earth is the water that is present in the uncooked, natural foods we consume. Vegetables are critical in staving off disease, so it is important to consider how you prepare your vegetables. "Raw" food is food that has not been heated to a temperature above 105 to 115 degrees Fahrenheit (depending upon which source you consult). This excludes all packaged foods that have been pasteurized, unless they are labeled "raw" or "cold pressed."

Typically, raw foods include fruits, vegetables, grains, nuts, and seeds, but can also comprise meat, eggs, seafood, and dairy products.

Before I learned the amazing benefits of raw food, I went vegetarian. It was not an easy decision, and it was one that I know now was not even necessary. But at the time I made the decision, after reading book upon book about the tremendous nutrient content of vegetables compared to the "evils" of meat, I thought it had to be all or nothing. In fact, I made the decision twice. The first time, I told my husband and my running partner, and they both provided me with a dozen reasons why it was not a good idea. So I put my decision on hold and continued reading.

The next time I decided to become a vegetarian, I kept it to myself. It was even harder to make the decision the second time around. I laid in bed for three days thinking about the monumental decision I was embarking on while I told those around me I wasn't feeling well. I had never experienced a dilemma so heavy; it weighed me down to the point that I couldn't get out of bed. By the third day though, I knew I wanted to be vegetarian, and I knew I would have to keep a lid on it.

The decision to go vegetarian was an important social learning experience. What I learned is that it is often best to keep new healthy lifestyle choices to yourself, at least initially. One reason is because you need to make these decisions for you and your health, not for anybody else. Another reason is that it is not uncommon for your friends and family to try to talk you out of healthy lifestyle transitions. It's not that they want to thwart your wellness, it's just that change can be difficult for people to accept, especially with regard to diet and lifestyle changes that they might not understand.

Originally I gave up meat and dairy, kept eggs, and added fish. Since then, I have allowed a little dairy, primarily in the form of cheese, and a very small amount of meat back into my diet. It should be noted though that the amount of cheese I eat has a direct impact on my weight; more cheese = higher weight. A quick fix is to stop eating cheese.

There is no right answer for everyone at every age at every time of year. What works for you today may completely change by next year. What you put into your mouth is up to you, and you can tweak it as needed as you go along. Nothing has to be in set in stone. Joshua Rosenthal, author of Integrative Nutrition, and founder of The Institute of Integrative Nutrition coined the term "bio-individuality" to describe the different and changing needs of individuals. What's important is that you recognize that what you put into your mouth does affect you health.

Thanks to another elderly neighbor, Mimi, raw

food entered my world about six months after I adopted my semi-vegetarian lifestyle. In 2010, at age 71, Mimi earned the title of "PETA's Sexiest Vegetarian over 50." When Mimi first began eating 100 percent raw food, she enthusiastically reported to me how much her energy increased and how satisfying the food was. That wasn't what convinced me raw food warranted further investigation though. I had lots of energy, which I assumed was because of my running, biking, and vegetarian diet. What convinced me that raw food was worth looking into was that Mimi's increased energy was concurrent with a lack of discussion about arthritic pain. Every older person I've ever known has been inclined to speak frequently about aches and pains. Mimi was no exception until a couple of months into her new diet regimen of 100 percent raw food.

Suddenly she was smiling all the time and speaking about how energized she felt; not similar to any 70-plus-year-old woman I've ever known. In addition, Mimi told me she had recently received high blood pressure and cholesterol lowering agent prescriptions from her doctor but both conditions and her arthritis resolved after she began eating 100% raw food. She never even filled the prescriptions.

Normalization of blood pressure and remittance of arthritic pain is a big deal. If I had been suffering from those problems at that time, I immediately would have jumped on the raw food bandwagon. It was Mimi's hair that convinced me of the value of a raw diet. Previously, Mimi's hair was more typical of older adults, but I witnessed it grow longer and thicker than I had ever seen it. It was hair that I, 22 years younger, would have loved to call my own.

Four years after she began her raw food journey, Mimi, now 75 years young, has published two raw food cookbooks: Live Raw and Live Raw Around the World. In addition, she has recently completed a third book on juicing: The Ultimate Book of Modern Juicing.

Before I read a single book on the subject, I was convinced that incorporating more raw foods into my own diet was the right thing to do.

Lately I have seen an outpouring of juicing books and detox agendas that involve vegetable juicing. The benefits are worth the buzz. It is simply the quickest and most efficient method of flooding your body with a smorgasbord of readily absorbable vital nutrients while at the same time providing your body with the perfectly pure sun-drenched hydration it needs to thrive. Drinking one 12- to 16-ounce glass of fresh vegetable juice and eating at least one large green salad every day will make it easy for you to consume the recommended daily allowance of vegetables.

I don't recommend substituting fruit in place of vegetables; vegetables are just too important.

Fruit should be consumed in addition to your five servings of vegetables, and they generally should not be juiced. Drinking fruit juice, like drinking soda, delivers too big of a sugar load straight to the liver without the fiber to slow the process; it throws homeostasis a curve ball. I frequently use fruit to curb those between-meal hunger pangs. Whole fruits are my version of "fast food" and are great to grab when you're on the way out the door. I always have a healthy snack in my purse to prevent inopportune hunger from derailing my intentions to eat right. Not that I don't ever eat things that aren't good for me — nobody is perfect — but if I'm going to eat unhealthful, at least I'm going to do it intentionally and not because it's all that's available.

Ancient Chinese medicine recommends 80 percent of one's daily calories should be obtained from raw foods, while western medical practitioners don't have a clue about the benefits of raw food. It was once thought that the active enzymes contained in raw or "live" foods were killed or inactivated by digestive juices. Dr. H. E. Kirschner in his 1957 book, Live Food Juices, describes multiple instances of using fresh vegetable juices to heal patients of a multitude of illnesses that left other doctors stumped. Unfortunately our conventional medical establishment still tends to purport as quackery all methods of health preservation that they don't explicitly provide (at a very high cost).

I kid you not, the rewards of increasing the amount of raw food in your diet is no scam. Do your own research on this topic by getting a routine physical health assessment and discussing with your doctor your plans to incorporate more raw foods into your diet (salads, juices, fruit, seeds, nuts). Then schedule a physical reassessment two or more months down the road, so you and your doctor can observe a marked reduction in your numerical stats (weight, cholesterol, blood pressure, C-reactive protein). When your doctor comments on the obvious beneficial changes, you can educate him or her about juicing and ancient Chinese wisdom.

Consuming large mounts of raw food can even prevent sunburn. I have blonde hair, blue eyes, and naturally fair skin. Living in sunny Southern California, I used to get sunburned on occasion, but no longer since I started making raw food a main stay of my diet. How? Think about it, sunburn is simply inflammation. Raw vegetables are anti-inflammatories.

If raw foods can prevent the inflammation that results from too much sun, what other causes of inflammation can they prevent? Since most disease is now known to be the result of excessive inflammation, obviously anti-inflammatory raw foods will be helpful in preventing most disease. It's all so darn simple, how can conventional medicine continue to get away with keeping us in the dark?

Yoga

Yoga was an important addition to my new healthy lifestyle thanks to Laura, my long-time biking and running partner. Laura is an avid yoga practitioner and credits it for enabling her to continue jogging. Some years back, Laura suffered from knee pain and was told she needed surgery and that even with surgery, she most likely would never be able to run again. Laura opted out of knee surgery and instead took a year off from running while she practiced yoga. That was nearly 12 years ago, during most of which she has been my workout partner. Ten- and 12-mile jaunts up Iron Mountain or Mt. Gower, usually just once a week, is my routine, but Laura has been doing it three or four times a week for the last 10 or 12 years. Laura's knee is just fine.

For years, I wanted to start practicing yoga myself, but I always felt awkward and out of place when I'd try a class. I also found yoga classes to be too expensive to do on a regular basis. Eventually a coworker hooked me up with a beginner's class at a yoga studio near the hospital where we worked. It was something my husband and I could do together (my running and biking is way out of his league), so we attended the 45-minute class every Friday. Not only did the yoga increase my strength and flexibility, it helped my marriage by giving my husband and I additional time together. We began having date nights every Friday after yoga. The euphoric feeling that comes after stretching with deep intentional breathing was a great way to start the evening.

In my late 40s, I realized I was practicing all the healthful lifestyle behaviors I learned about as a kid watching that 60 Minutes segment. All except one — meditation still was not part of my routine until I read a short book about it at 2:00 a.m. one night when I couldn't sleep midway through a ten-day master cleanse. After finishing the book, I immediately felt myself descending into oblivion and had a very surreal dream. Exactly one hour later I awoke with the idea of writing a book about health and the crazy, mixed-up medical establishment, buoyed by an inner peace and confidence that meditation would guide me. Now whenever I arrive at a destination early, I stay in my car and use the extra time to meditate.

Even if exercise and more water and vegetables have not yet made their way into your daily routine, I urge you to try meditation. Meditation is just a fancy way of giving yourself a little space in time to sit quietly and breathe. Five or ten minutes is all it takes. You can take a class or read a book to help aid you in your meditative journey, but no matter what you desire, if you're not meeting your desired goals or dreams, meditation can help.

Earthing

Another free-and-easy practice that you can work into your regular routine is called "earthing" or "grounding." Earthing involves skin-to-skin contact with the ground. Our bodies are electrical systems, and every biochemical reaction is electrical in nature. The Earth is like a giant battery continually being recharged by radiation from the sun. When the Earth and a human body are in direct contact, without the impedance of nonconductive materials such as rubber, plastic, wood, or glass, an exchange of electrons occurs that helps regulate the body's biologic electrical systems. Simply walking barefoot on the bare ground can make a positive contribution to your body's efforts to achieve and maintain balance.

There are specialized pads and mattresses you can purchase that plug into the grounding access of electrical sockets and deliver constant electrical current from the Earth while you sleep. One thing I like about earthing though is that you don't have to purchase anything to take advantage of this wellness strategy. It's free and available to all. I make a point of taking my shoes off at parks and at the beach whenever I can. Shoes, pavement, and other building materials act as barriers that cut us off from the natural healing power of the Earth

Studies demonstrate that 30- to 40 minutes of direct skin-to-Earth contact prevents inflammation and blood clotting, which are the very causes of numerous disease conditions the pharmaceutical industry is making a killing on. The answer has been under our feet all along (Earthing, Ober, Sinatra, Zucker, 2010).

Chapter 5: Beauty Comes from Within

Beauty is inherent. I'm not just talking about spiritual beauty, I mean the kind we see with our eyes: clear, smooth skin; rosy cheeks; thicker, stronger hair; and straight teeth. Men and women of every age the world over spend billions of dollars on beauty products in an effort to achieve a perceived vision of good looks. Combine this with the money spent on cosmetic procedures and the beauty industry is probably second only to the medical industry in terms of dollars spent.

What if you knew that the same things that make you healthy on the inside show up on the outside as clear, smooth skin; rosy cheeks; thicker, stronger hair; and straight teeth. Yes, our health and nutritional status (and that of our parents) even plays a role in the alignment of our teeth. Weston Price's study of nutrition and teeth demonstrated that the more a civilization's diet stayed close to its ancestral past, untainted by the industrial food machine, whether plant or animal based, the prettier their smiles and more symmetrical their faces.

Speaking of pretty smiles and faces, the lovely models used in the world of advertising are not only promoting the product they are selling, they are also championing societal norms of beauty. It is apparent that our culture places great value on being thin, yet, ironically, if we consume the junk foods these models are promoting, there is no way we could attain this vision of perfection. Nearly all advertised foods are either "fast foods" or highly processed foods, both of which are harmful to health and physical appearance.

Likewise, the beautiful middle-age men and women advertising the vast array of pharmaceutical products do not in the least resemble the typical chronically ill patients I care for and who use these types of products. In advertising, perception is reality, but in the real world, the world I see every day, the reality is aged and decrepit bodies ruined by unhealthy foods and medicines. Drug advertisements that use beautiful, thin people to promise the miraculous cessation of a variety of symptoms for dozens of different ailments while gentle music plays in the background are for substances that purportedly "manage" medical problems. What they don't tell you is that these medical problems would likely not exist if you drank water, walked, ate vegetables, and meditated on a regular basis.

Doctors should be prescribing water, vegetables, exercise, and meditation. This is the type of information that needs to be driven home to our children and young people, who have been raised on dangerous, chemically laden food. They need to know why the shapes of their bodies do not match those found in all those advertisements and why their skin frequently looks like a combat zone. Everyone must learn that junk food manufacturers and drug producers make quite a bit of money selling their products, but their products make us fat, ugly, disabled, and miserable.

On the other hand, supplying your body with nutrient-rich foods containing vitamins and other micronutrients keeps you feeling and looking younger. I personally notice a more radiant and glowing complexion within minutes of drinking a green vegetable juice drink. Sometimes when I look in the mirror and see a pale, sallow me look back, I say to myself, "you need some green juice." When I ready myself for a special occasion, preparing a green juice drink is as important to me as bathing and dressing up.

While on the subject of beauty, I must again mention raw food and Mimi, the now 75-year-old sexy vegan who got me started. Raw food has been said to "youth" you (the opposite of "aging" you). It seems to be working for Mimi. Like most people, I love desserts and snacks, but traditional goodies don't promote health. Raw bars and pies are healthful and guiltless. Preparing raw desserts and snacks has enabled me to consume healthful, organic, raw vegan treats — I can have my "cake" and eat it too.

While on a recent train trip to Seattle to visit family on Orcas Island, I couldn't help but notice what other people on the train were eating. It is apparent that Americans believe vacations and road trips are an excuse to ditch one's regular diet in exchange for convenient out-of-a-bag, crunchy, salty snacks. All around me, young and old alike were consuming Cheetos, potato chips, crackers, and the like with gusto. They taste good and they travel well, no doubt, and we have to eat, don't we?

Actually, we don't. Our bodies are better off experiencing a bit of hunger rather than being inundated with a mess of snacks that don't in the slightest way resemble real food. Not only do our bodies perform quite well for many hours without food, there are health benefits to resting the digestive system by skipping a meal or two or even several. The Miracle of Fasting by Paul Bragg describes many of these health benefits, including one that I find extremely supportive of a long and healthy life: fasting helps prevent and cure metabolic syndrome, possibly by helping to rid the liver of excess fat created by consuming too much sugar. Our ancient ancestors routinely benefitted from fasting, because food wasn't always available. Logically, it seems that fasting forces your body to burn stored fat (from the liver or hips) and as long as you have plenty to spare, this is a good thing.

Despite the benefits of fasting, my husband and I did not go hungry on that 36-hour train trip. I had a stash of treats big enough to last us a week, most of them homemade, raw, and vegan. I made granola, nutty fruit bars, and my old standby, chocolate-chip cookies (to fulfill my craving for chocolate). Together with two large salads stored in a personal cooler, the same cooler I use to store my packed lunch at work, my husband and I had plenty of healthy food to share on our two-day train ride.

Making bars and cookies from raw ingredients and using a dehydrator instead of an oven takes no more "active" time than the preparation of conventional cookies.

1. Throw all the ingredients in a bowl and stir.
2. Spread the batter on a cookie sheet.
3. Pop it in the oven or dehydrator.
4. Wait for them to cook.

Pretty easy, huh? The main difference is the length of time you wait before your creation is ready to be enjoyed. Oh yeah, and the amazing health benefits.

I find the batter or dough of raw preparations tastes more like the finished product compared to conventionally cooked foods, so if what you've put together tastes good undone, it will taste the same, just dryer and crunchier after a few or several hours of dehydrating at 105 degrees Fahrenheit. Like any type of baking or cooking, it just takes some practice figuring out when its done.

For bars and cookie treats, I like this method:

1. Soak a combination of nuts, seeds, and grains in water overnight. Rinse and drain.
2. Place one to two cups of soaked nuts (almonds, pecans, and/or walnuts) in a very powerful blender (like a Vita Mix) along with one to two cups of soaked sunflower seeds and one to two cups of soaked flax seeds and one to two cups of soaked grains (barley, quinoa, and/or oats).
3. (Optional) Add a handful of soaked dates (minus the pits) or other ripe fruit to add sweetness including bananas, apples, persimmons, pomegranates, figs, and so on.
4. Add one-half to one full cup of honey for desired sweetness.
5. Blend till smooth and place batter in a large mixing bowl.
6. Add all the chopped nuts, raisins, chocolate chips, and chopped fresh or dried fruits you desire.
7. (Optional) To increase the richness of the finished product, add peanut butter or almond butter.
8. (Optional) Mix in a pinch of salt and a few drops of vanilla.

A big batch of this will fill up several dehydrator sheets, making literally dozens of servings. I score them into bars before dehydrating, which makes it easier to cut them into bars later. They store well long term in the refrigerator in sealed containers and also travel well when refrigeration is not available.

Many of the ingredients listed here are optional, but what are not optional are the flax seeds, which provide a stickiness that holds the whole lot together. One time I was following a recipe for making crackers out of mostly bell peppers and carrot pulp. The batter tasted wonderful, and I was expecting a spicy Mexican-flavored cracker. Unfortunately the recipe didn't call for flax seeds or any other sticky gooey substance (chia seeds also work), and while dehydrating, my crackers dried into a lovely mess of tiny orange granules that I ended up using as popcorn seasoning. Lesson learned.

Eating these kinds of snacks, along with a salad, fresh fruit, and a green vegetable drink, keeps me going all day during my 12-hour shifts at the hospital. They also keep blemishes away and keep my weight down. Most important, my primarily whole foods diet — rich in raw vegetables and low in processed foods — helps prevent the development of "chronic" illness.

Chapter 6: Love and Death

Death is never convenient. Few of us are ever prepared to deal with the ramifications a fatal diagnosis brings. But early premature death is the hardest to swallow.

Raphael

Raphael and I first met at the El Cajon, California, courthouse on July 3, 2013. He was there to see the court facilitator about the divorce his wife had filed for in June. I was there in an attempt to end alimony payments from a divorce of my own from 10 years previous. Our conversation started because I overheard him say he had cancer and wouldn't be around forever, which was why he didn't understand his wife's choices.

I interrupted to offer some morale support about his divorce, and then asked him what he was doing about the cancer. He crossed the distance between us and sat down next to me, and for the next 90 minutes, we discussed everything under the sun related to health. Before we parted, we learned much about each other, including that we both lived in the small town of Ramona. Raphael told me about his job as a web designer and business manager. I told him that I was a nurse who very much wanted to start a new business promoting health, and I needed help building a website. I offered to make him "green drinks" in exchange for assistance with web design, and we agreed to get together after my upcoming Fourth of July camping trip.

Two weeks passed, and I had pretty much given up hope Raphael would contact me. Then, the day before I left on another trip — a 10-day trip to Orcas Island, Washington, to visit family — his call came. I agreed to meet with him that afternoon.

Raphael was living at Dan's house, a paraplegic wheelchair-bound friend and member of his church. Rafael's wife had kicked him out of their home three months after his diagnosis.

I noted Raphael's skin had lightened since our courthouse meeting; at that time it displayed the dark hue of a person with liver disease. Now his skin appeared normal, not diseased. I also noted Raphael's abdomen was slimmer; at our first meeting I had noted a moderately enlarged middle. He told me he used to be significantly overweight but changes he made to help rid his body of cancer, including his recent vegetarian diet and the addition of regular exercise, were benefitting his waistline, too.

Raphael was Mormon and it was important for him to make it understood at the start that our relationship was to remain platonic. I of course was married, and we agreed to maintain a business relationship that was to revolve around our mutual passion for health and helping people to achieve it. He showed me the website he was working on called Heal My Cancer Now and told me he wanted me to be a part of it. Because I was an RN, he believed my input would give the site credibility as an informative health source.

In addition to transforming to a nearly vegan diet and bicycling, Raphael had just began using a machine he recently purchased that emitted sound waves directly at the cancerous liver tumors. He was excited to share this with me.

Like at the courthouse, time passed quickly and we never ran out of things to talk about. I agreed to contact him as soon as I got back from my trip. After my return in early August, we met three or four times before he subjected himself, at his doctor's recommendation, to his first (and last) dose of chemo on August 14, 2013. Just one week prior to the chemo, a CT scan demonstrated his liver tumor was smaller, and Raphael's doctor said his liver function was good. I still have the excited voicemail he left me on my cell phone giving me the good news.

At our meetings, we discussed a book I wanted to write. Raphael wanted to help me. He told me about his plans to turn the land around the home where he was living into an organic farm. With each meeting, our book project progressed. He put up poster board and worked with colored markers as he picked both our brains for book material. He even came up with a working title and designed a cover for my book, taping it to the sliding glass door to inspire us while we worked.

While working on the book and sharing our personal stories, a deep friendship evolved. After just a few visits, I couldn't imagine not knowing Raphael. The fact that he had been diagnosed with liver cancer five months previously (with a prognosis of just six to nine months to live) wasn't relevant, because he didn't look sick and he was so clear about his plans for the future. In fact, each time we met he appeared slimmer and stronger, and he told me his bike rides along the paved roads of Ramona were getting longer.

Though the book we were corroborating on was about the confused medical system and its reliance on pharmaceuticals and chemical treatments, Raphael told me he planned to have a device implanted on August 14, 2013, that would be used to administer chemo. I didn't think it was a good idea—I tend to oppose medical procedures in general, and I really hate chemo, which poisons the body along with the cancer. Because I had only known Raphael a short time, I didn't think it my place to tell him what he should or shouldn't do, especially since I couldn't guarantee that green vegetable juice and a vegan diet were going to cure him.

It was supposed to be just a 20-minute procedure requiring one night in the hospital. I hoped I would be able change Rafael's mind about getting the chemo treatment before his appointment in six weeks. Little did I know (I am not convinced that Raphael even knew) it was chemo, not a device, he was to receive on that fateful day.

On August 14, 2013, the day of Raphael's scheduled procedure, Laura, my usual biking and running partner, was not available, so I invited Raphael to bike with me. He arrived promptly at 7:00 a.m. and we went for a 1.5-hour ride that included one steep hill and a couple of moderate hills with miles of flat roads interspersed between. Back at my house, I juiced green drinks of cilantro, celery, beets, carrots, and green apple for both of us.

Halfway done with his green drink, Raphael received the call from Mercy Hospital that he had been expecting. They had a bed ready, and he could come in right away. We talked for another 30 minutes while we drank our breakfast; I secretly hoped he'd miss his procedure. Raphael was ready to go though. I asked permission to come see him in the hospital, and he agreed I could come by later that afternoon after it was over. I would be his only visitor, because the doctor had assured him it would be just a one-night stay in the hospital and he could drive himself home the next day.

When I visited him later that day, he appeared healthy and happy, good as new — all was well. Or so it seemed. The following morning when I texted to inquire about his release, things had changed. He had gotten faint and hypotensive after his shower that morning and internal bleeding was suspected. Later in the day, Raphael was moved to the ICU. My distrust of western medicine and their use of poisons and sharp instruments grew.

Raphael's expected one-night stay in the hospital turned into almost a week. After six days in the ICU, on Monday, he was told that he would most likely be released at the end of the week. Instead, he was abruptly released Tuesday afternoon, the fallowing day. In fact, he was wheeled out to the curb, where he managed to get a security guard to help him find his car.

Rafael was in no shape to go home or to drive. His abdomen had grown from a size 38 to a size 46 during his six-day hospitalization, and he was unsteady on his feet. Raphael was returning to a home where he had no one to assist him with meals or to help him to the bathroom, assistance he did not require the day he entered the hospital, the day he went bike riding with me.

I became Raphael's meal preparer, but he had no appetite. It took hours for him to consume a few bites of eggs or rice. He could not even stomach the green drinks I filled his fridge with. Before, when we met to work on our business plans, we always sat outside, but it took Raphael four days after being discharged and driving himself home from Mercy Hospital before he had the strength to walk to the front door. On more than one occasion, I witnessed him crawl to the bathroom on his hands and knees. He wouldn't allow me to assist him because he was concerned it would necessitate inappropriate physical contact.

Ten days later, Raphael had a follow-up appointment with his oncologist. I offered to drive him — I had a few questions for the doctor. At the appointment, I learned Rafael did not have a device for administering chemo inserted in his body on August 14. Instead, Raphael had received transcatheter arterial chemoembolization (TACE). TACE is an interventional radiological procedure that punctures the common femoral artery in the right groin and threads a catheter through the abdominal aorta and through the celiac trunk and common hepatic artery to the branch of the proper hepatic artery supplying blood to the tumor; chemo is channeled through the catheter and released directly to the tumor (http://en.wikipedia.org/wiki/Transcatheter_arterial_chemoembolization). The oncologist said there was no systemic circulation of the chemo; it only went to the tumor. My distrust of western medicine increased — no human can control what enters the body's circulatory system and prevent if from circulating throughout the rest of the body, not even one possessing a medical degree.

The oncologist explained that the bleeding that had resulted in two days in critical care was "the largest tumor dying off," and that later treatments would most likely not go so badly because the other tumors were smaller. I could not believe she thought Rafael should have this treatment again! Of course, the doctor was just saying what she thought Rafael wanted to hear. She actually had no way of knowing what was going on with the tumors on Raphael's liver because no follow-up CT scans had been done. Later, when follow-up CT scans were performed, they revealed the tumor had grown and spread (though this information was withheld from Raphael until much later).

In my opinion, the oncologist was providing information that only God could have known, and it is this matter-of-fact, know-it-all attitude often displayed by medical doctors that convinces the general public that the doctor knows best. In reality, doctors learn their craft at medical schools, where slicing, dicing, and prescribing are the curriculum. It is what they know best.

What they don't learn in medical school is the natural healing ability of the body when it is provided with an abundance of nutrients.

Raphael learned after his diagnosis that cancer was more likely to develop in those with sedentary lifestyles and diets lacking vegetables and rich in animal products and sugar. In the five months between his diagnosis and his chemotherapy, he had made the necessary changes in attempt to reverse cancer.

And it had been working. His oncologist had failed to recognize that Raphael's progress during those five months was an obvious sign that the cancer in his body was well controlled. The CT scan taken before his chemo treatment revealed that Raphael's body was successfully managing the cancer without succumbing to it, and his doctor's medical advice should have been to keep doing what he was doing.

Raphael, age 57, now appeared 30 years older than he had when we went cycling on August 14, and he was having difficulty positioning himself on the examining table. Yet the doctor recommended more chemo treatments! Raphael left the appointment with a prescription for Lasix, a powerful diuretic that was supposed to help him with his bloated abdomen, otherwise known as ascites.

Ascites usually develops in patients with chronic liver failure because albumin, a protein normally manufactured by the liver that helps maintain oncotic pressure, is not being produced. Without albumin, fluid leaks out of blood vessels and is deposited wherever it can find space. This causes edema (swelling) of the peritoneum, the cavity that houses the abdominal organs. As fluid accumulates, it causes the abdomen to expand, resembling a woman's pregnant belly.

In Raphael's case, I believe the bleeding into his abdomen, along with the toxic chemo he received, resulted in severe inflammation throughout his abdominal cavity and a sudden onset of severe ascites. This was a huge burden to him after leaving the hospital; his mobility was limited and his clothes didn't fit.

That evening, Raphael received a call from his oncologist informing him that she was not going to be his doctor anymore, something to do with insurance she said. It seemed to both of us that she either quit the case or was fired by the powers that be because she messed him up so badly.

The Lasix didn't help, even after the dose was doubled. Raphael didn't get better and after a couple weeks struggling at home with increased pain and decreased mobility, he texted me at work and informed me he was calling 911 to go back to the hospital. He was admitted to Pomerado Hospital in Poway, where they performed a paracentesis procedure, draining five liters of ascitic fluid from his bloated abdomen.

A follow-up CT was performed and it revealed an enlarged liver tumor that had spread. Raphael though was not informed of this information, and his new oncologist told him that the TACE procedure was a bad choice for Raphael and he would not be recommending any more TACE treatments.

A week later, he transferred to Vibra Hospital in Hillcrest because that's where his health insurance - Medi-Cal - was willing to pay for him to be. After his transfer to Vibra, I spent every day off at his bedside, bringing him food and drink (that mostly went uneaten), taking pictures of him for evidence of what chemo wrought, and getting to know and respect this intelligent and kind human being.

Over the next five weeks Raphael remained at Vibra. While tending to him in the hospital or at his house, I met his sister, Margarita, who came out from Nashville, his brother, Alan, sister-in-law, Ofelia, and his mother, who lived locally in San Marcos. Though at first I was unsure of how his family would receive me, a stranger to them, they immediately put me at ease, telling me repeatedly that I was an angel sent from heaven to be with Rafael during this unfortunate time in his life.

I also met several members of Raphael's Mormon Church community who made the trip down the hill from Ramona to see Raphael during his various hospital stays. Through them I learned of Raphael's volunteer work coaching basketball and home teaching. It became obvious to me how well respected he was among the church leaders and congregation.

Raphael and I looked at Facebook pictures of his family while he lovingly told me about his five children, four daughters and one son ranging in ages from 10 to 20. We read about Colombia, Raphael's place of birth, on my laptop computer and listened to Colombian music. Raphael told me he wanted to go back one day to visit when he was well. He hadn't visited in years. We also played backgammon on Rafael's notebook computer, a gift from Margarita. We spent a great deal of time attempting to write about Raphael's horrific ordeal and having no idea how it was going to end.

On September 19, 2013, I visited Raphael at Vibra hospital. Sitting in a chair next to his bed, feeling the warm sun on my face, I considered all that my friend had been through. It had been one month and five days since the TACE procedure, and Raphael had not improved. His abdomen was still large and round, his color yellowish brown, and he required a walker to go to the bathroom. He told me that his biggest regret in life was allowing the medical establishment to have its way with him. He still believed he would get better in time, but felt the last month had been a waste of his precious time. He had a business to run and was anxious for this period in his life to pass so he could get on with it.

It was very hard to take. Rafael was doing fine when I met him back on that July afternoon at the courthouse. For a man who had been given six to nine months to live just five months previously, he was eating well, exercising, and feeling and looking better than he had in years. And then came the chemo.

The following day, Margarita returned home to Nashville. She has been in San Diego bringing food and good thoughts and prayers to Raphael's bedside for four weeks. While in San Diego, she led and joined women from Raphael's church, his sister-in-law Ofelia, and his mother for a housecleaning party to tidy up Dan's house and Raphael's bedroom. After Margarita left, Raphael was discharged, and I drove him home from Vibra Hospital to his newly cleaned and decorated home.

On the way home from Vibra Hospital, Raphael wanted to stop at the beach and soak his feet in the ocean. Sadly, he could only muster the strength to drag his new walker to the sand at the edge of the parking lot at Ocean Beach pier. It was great seeing him outside though, and I have some nice pictures of the event. Raphael had ventured outside only twice while at Vibra Hospital, both times to the outdoor patio area that doubled as the staff smoking spot.

Unfortunately, it was too smoky for Raphael to tolerate, but he would not let me complain about it because he didn't want to impose on others. That's the kind of man he was.

When we got to his house, Raphael's eyes filled with tears upon seeing what others had done for him. He was to enjoy his new space for less than two weeks before returning to Pomerado Hospital. During that short time I was able to take Raphael on two field trips. We went to lunch one rainy afternoon at Thai Time, a new Thai restaurant in Ramona. I will never forget Rafael's smiling face as he sat across from me at our table next to the window wrapped in his purple blanket (he didn't own a coat that fit his new post-chemo body) while rain poured outside. The food was great and so was the company.

Our second outing was lunch at Chipotle restaurant in Santee, after which we went to see the movie Gravity with my youngest son, Zach. The movie was intense, and afterward Rafael told me his stomach was tight because of it. The tautness didn't end when the movie did though; it remained hard as a rock.

Though he had been discharged, Raphael was still bloated, using a walker, and lacking appetite as a result of chemo. To this day, I still do not know whether or not he knew he was getting the TACE treatment. I do know that he had no idea about the ramifications of chemo, especially where liver cancer is concerned.

Chemo is especially dangerous for patients with liver cancer, because the liver is the primary detoxifying organ in the body. Any chemo you receive is going to be filtered through the liver further stressing an already impaired organ. The fact that he was doing so well five months into his diagnosis, as demonstrated by his blood work, CT scans, and physical appearance and mobility, that the medical community opted to intervene, is a crime, in my opinion.

Not long after that, Raphael called 911, once again for unmanaged pain. I saw him at his home on my way back from work that day, and some time during the night he was transported to Pomerado Hospital. He texted me when he was in the ER, and the following morning I left for work early so I could stop for a quick visit on my way before my shift started at Palomar Hospital. He was asleep when I walked in the room. I sat down next to him and he awoke. We both cried.

His second paracentesis was done the following day, and this time, more than six liters of fluid were removed. The plan was for Rafael to be discharged the following day with hospital equipment, including a hospital bed and subcutaneous pain medication infusion in place that could be managed as needed by Raphael and hospice care. The involvement of hospice care meant Raphael was going home with the expectation of death within six months. He finally was informed of his CT scan results indicating the spread of the liver tumors into his peritoneal cavity.

Raphael lasted only two days. He died on October 28, 2013; just two months and 12 days after his one and only chemo treatment. His brother and I took turns being with him after his final release. Alan took the night shift and I the day shift. His soon-to-be ex-wife and their children stayed with him during the evening as well. His two oldest daughters travelled by bus from Utah and arrived in the wee hours of the morning, just hours before Raphael passed.

I am grateful for the time I was given with this special human being, and I will forever wonder if western medicine is capable of recognizing the error of its ways.

Mom

Following is my sister Evelyn's recollection of our Mom's end of life.

In May 2006, I received a call from Mom. This call was different than usual. Mom seemed anxious, concerned that she may have a serious medical problem. It was especially clear in Mom's voice, though she tried to hide it, that I needed to visit her before her next doctor appointment. I dropped everything and checked the ferry schedule. The next boat was due to leave in about an hour and one-half. I threw a few things in a bag, called my husband, Mike, and left.

When I got to the ferry, they were turning everyone away. Ferries at that time of year are often overloaded, and it's just something you have to deal with. This time it wasn't OK though. I had to go, I was not going to be turned away. It was an emergency. My mother needed me.

Up to this point, I'd been handling the day like a champ. But there was no way in hell I was going to miss this ferry. I had to get to my mother. Suddenly I cracked, my emotions collapsed, and I begged the poor ticket handler to allow me on the ferry so I could get to my mom as quickly as possible. I instinctively knew Mom was in fear her life was going to be cut short, and I couldn't allow any obstacle to keep us apart.

Mom was never one to ask for help, but thankfully I have always been able to sense her need. By some people's standards, my mom was not an amazing mother. But I have a different set of criteria. I see her as a simple, undemanding woman who had eleven children and umpteen grandchildren and loved them all more than life. She suffered and enjoyed. She deserved every possible thing life could bring, especially my love, every bit of it. I certainly had not been an easy child for her, ever, and still she loved me and trusted me, even at a time like this. I was ready to raise hell or high water, whatever she needed, to be there for her at that moment. Let's just say they let me on that ferry and leave it at that.

The first night I got there we lay in bed together and talked about what the doctor had told her. She had been dropping quite a bit of weight during the year, and now a mass had been discovered on her pancreas. We discussed how she wanted to cope with it, if it was cancer, and how she could accept this fate and be comforted by her faith. Even with a strong faith though, who is ever really ready to accept this ultimate sentence? Mom and I kept it pretty light that first night, then the next day my sister Rachelle arrived.

Mom was so thin that her clothes hung off her, so we took her shopping and bought some really nice outfits and then went out for a nice dinner. We had a great time. The next day, the three of us went together to her doctor appointment.

After 15 minutes in the waiting room, we were ushered in to see the doctor. Right off the bat, we got hit with it: tests are conclusive, it's pancreatic cancer, chances are, maybe, six months. Get your shit in order. Sorry, there's nothing we can do for you.

Mom didn't complain much about her pain, she

never did. Her pain tolerance was high. She insisted that eating made her uncomfortable though, unless it was a jelly donut. No complaint there.

In the following days, there was a very uncomfortable lack of direction. What to do next? There is no direction given to the dying. The patient is ordained with terminal cancer, and then what? Maybe go insane? Thank God for the Internet. I got online and found a cancer center in Seattle, one that treated pancreatic cancer. A call to them confirmed that yes, although expensive — $8000 per month — they could see Mom. She was grateful to have the ongoing support of a doctor.

This is a woman that worships the almighty MD. I was relieved that Mom might find some comfort but also very worried about the cost. How the heck were we going to pay for it? Never mentioned that one to Mom, except to say, "don't worry about that Mom, it will be handled."

Mom was excited to get started right away with treatment; she would have done anything to get better. It was a busy time. I almost completely stopped working in order to be with Mom. We paid our bills with borrowed money. Thank God we had a credit line on our house.

Mom moved in with us. We stayed at our house on Orcas Island Friday night to Tuesday morning, when we would take the ferry to Anacortes. Mom had a medical priority loading status for the ferry, which she loved dearly, bless her heart. We got to drive down to the front of the line every Tuesday morning. We were always the first to get on, right up front with the best view on the boat as we journeyed to the cancer center in Seattle. Tuesday was chemotherapy day. It was always a nice drive, a nice visit, a political and socioeconomic recess of everything that was wrong and how to fix it. We would stop at the Safeway near the center and get a drink and a donut for Mom and an espresso for me before heading over for her 11:00 a.m. appointment.

The people at the cancer center were wonderful. They really supported Mom's will to live, attacking her illness with mind, body, and soul support. She would see two or three doctors and then have her chemotherapy. The sessions lasted from one to three hours every week. On Tuesday nights, we took it easy, often stopping for a light dinner as we headed to Mom's condo in Bellingham for the night, sometimes two.

I wanted to make sure Mom didn't loose touch with what she knew. She loved her home, family, and friends. On Wednesdays and sometimes Thursdays, she welcomed visitors. I used this time to take care of her bills and banking, which gave me a little respite.

I really think in spite of everything, Mom enjoyed this time. She knew that we were going to be together from then on and that it was going to be OK, a sentiment that I encouraged. We had fun together. We really did. On Thursday nights, we headed back to the island with Mom proudly taking her position at the front of the ferry line. She loved it. She would always say, "It's good to be going home." She loved it there on Orcas Island, where she knew she belonged and could relax.

That is until the night she fell in the bathroom. My daughter Sam came and woke me up, "Grandma fell in the bathroom and I can't pick her up." I went to the bathroom and Mom was lying on the floor. She said with something between a cry and a chuckle, " I can't get up." Sam held her hand, and I picked her up. She only weighed about 125 pounds, despite her five-foot, nine-inch frame.

I walked her back to her room and stayed with her that night. She seemed fine and slept. The next morning, my husband, Mike, called his local doctor and asked him to see Mom. He came right over and continued to see her once or twice a week. He was always kind enough to see Mom at home. I called my siblings. Mom had really taken a turn for the worse. The doctor felt she was in the best place she could be. Apparently she had suffered a stroke and was close to death.

Mike had grown accustomed to lifting Mom by this time, God love him. He took great care with Mom, cooked her wonderful food, and patiently supported me while I spent every waking and sleeping hour with her. He even moved her into the master bedroom until the local hospice folks located a nice hospital bed for her to use. This gave Mom two beds in her room. She especially liked the one next to the window, where she could watch the fairies in the garden devour the juice of the Himalayan honeysuckle bushes outside. This floored her.

The hardest thing for Mom was accepting that she was pretty much bedridden and had to use a potty chair, which she hated. The doctor, two nurses, and a physical therapist made regular visits, supporting her in any way they could. I got up with her in the mornings and wheeled her into the shower in my room; thank God we had a wheelchair-accessible shower. She didn't like being showered at first, but as with everything, she adjusted.

After a few weeks of steady improvement, she asked me when we were going back to the cancer center for her next dose of chemo. Oh my, that was hard for me to answer. When I had called to cancel her last appointment, I was advised that she should not come back unless she regained her strength and health completely. They believed her chemo was the likely cause of her failing health. Now I had to tell her that we could not go back until she was fully recuperated and walking again. She cried, and I was so sorry.

Mom's illness was taking a toll on her whole body and her emotions. She became short-tempered, and that brought back memories of being young in Mom's house. This time around, however, I never took anything she said to heart. I knew she was suffering from failing health, was scared of dying, and was angry about the whole situation. We got through it thanks to the help and support of a wonderful family.

Shortly thereafter, Mom died in our home on Orcas Island.

Mom wasn't a heroic mother by any means. She didn't receive a lot of what she had needed when she was young. But she was a mother who loved and a grandmother whom everyone loved dearly. Since becoming a grandmother myself, there have been many times I've thought about how much she would have enjoyed her great-grandson, Gavin. I am sorry for anything that I have failed to provide my own children, and I pray they recognize, like I have about my mom, that I gave what I had. I will be eternally grateful for my mother, who I will always remember and love.

****

Mom lived to her mid 70's. Not long considering she worked right up until she was able to retire at age 65 (as many of us do). Like many of us, the last several years were not in the best of health - filled with prescriptions and doctor appointments. Certainly not the vibrancy that Mimi Kirk is experiencing today.

Chapter 7: Health Care of the Future

It wasn't long ago that western-trained physicians told women formula was better than the breast milk when it came to feeding their infants. The American Heart Association formerly encouraged Americans to eat margarine instead of butter because it was better than the real thing. Doctors used to sell cigarettes on TV.

Knowing that the majority of patients I've cared for over the years became ill because they failed to develop some simple tools for self-care is disconcerting, but working in a healthcare system that fails or even refuses to provide them with the tools of self-care is malpractice. It's time we human beings stopped sacrificing our health to the arrogance of mankind and start nourishing our bodies using healing strategies from nature.

Common sense dictates that we shouldn't be making or distorting our food in a science lab. Whether feeding your baby or yourself, it just makes sense to keep it natural. But don't be fooled by the term natural when it is displayed on a food product label. It means nothing other than the food industry's attempt to fool you into believing a product is safe for you and your family to consume. Let me tell you: their products are not safe if they are laden with sugar, table salt, MSG, or any other added ingredients that upset your body's biochemistry.

One of our body's methods for dealing with alien chemical additives is by sequestering them safely away in between layers of fat cells. This produces an internal drive to over consume. In other words, our bodies "naturally" fatten us up to provide a safety net against these toxins. Combined with the marketing hardball pitched at us daily by the food and pharmaceutical industries that manufacture deadly poisons, including food additives methodologically orchestrated to make sure you are never satiated, this makes it hard for people to find the healthy path.

Authentic natural foods are ones that have actually been grown in the ground and that satisfy your hunger without driving you to overeat. They come in a variety of natural colors but no artificial ones. No ingredients list is required on their packaging because they are what they appear to be; in fact, authentic natural foods need no packaging. If you don't want to go through life joined at the hip to the medical establishment, these foods should form the main part in your diet.

The medical community has a lot to answer for in not standing up for patients and providing the real scoop on maintaining and achieving wellness. Hippocrates, the so-called father of western medicine, would be disappointed with the modern state of health care. The apple has rolled far, far from the tree of life. The medical establishment has deemed you and I incapable of caring for our bodies the way nature intended, hoping we don't notice that what they offer is doing us more harm than good.

The United States ranks 37th in the world in quality of health care because our healthcare system has failed to recognize the facts of health. It has mistakenly removed self-health from the equation and duped us all into believing doctors know best. Enough is known about the harm sugar and excess animal protein does to the human body and about the benefits of vegetables and omega-3 supplementation, yet the unhealthy beat goes on. The current medical establishment has hindered the natural pursuit of good health long enough. Decades of proclaiming there is not enough proof or there have not been enough double-blind studies to validate any treatment or healing method that doesn't directly provide profit is not science, it's not medicine, it's pulling the wool over our eyes. Nutrition research indicates that whole foods are more effective than pharmaceuticals in keeping people healthy, and whole foods heal without harm. To hold back this information any longer is denying people the right to health and the pursuit of happiness

During my personal health journey, I couldn't help but notice that what I learned about the best ways to prevent disease was in direct opposition to my professional experience working in a hospital setting where ice cream, pies, cakes, and cookies are served up at every hospital celebratory function. Where numerous small packages of condiments containing artificial flavors and high-fructose corn syrup are served on every meal tray and where unnatural industrial liquid-food formulas are administered through nasogastric tubes to vulnerable patients. This unnatural nourishment that is disruptive to the healing process is the norm at most hospitals. It shouldn't be. These so called foods certainly shouldn't be the diet of choice when attempting to recover from illness.

I firmly believe that health or lack thereof is a direct result of what we put into our mouths on a daily basis. People look to hospitals as sources of healing and recovery. They should be role models for healthy food and habits, not places that encourage foods that foster disease.

In light of an epidemic of food- and lifestyle-related illness, not to mention jaw-dropping healthcare costs, it's time doctors and healthcare institutions made some changes. More effort and focus should be placed on educating patients and staff about the abundance of scientific information that is available about maintaining health and overcoming illness through diet. When the medical industry starts taking nutrition seriously then maybe the rest of the population will too. If hospital vending machines and cafeterias offered no artificial colors or preservatives, no GMOs, no hormones, and no antibiotics but instead served real food to patients and staff, not only would patients heal quicker, staff and their families might learn the value of food. A "No junk food" policy is paramount for teaching the community how valuable food is in preventing disease.

I must give credit where credit is due. Palomar Health, where I've worked the last 18 years, is starting to make some of these changes. Though their health-promoting program is in the very early stages, organic produce is now offered along with grass-fed and finished meat sources. Meatless Mondays are promoted as well as a "Rethink your drink" campaign to encourage beverages with less sugar. Physical activity is encouraged through computer health programs available to interested staff. Palomar Health has a long way to go to meet my expectations of what a healthcare environment should look like, but the fact that some of these changes are finally being made gives me hope that we're headed in the right direction. It's a signal to everybody that these types of diet modifications are credible and beneficial.

Historically, the AMA has squelched "alternative" health information by labeling it "quackery." In the age of the Internet though, they can no longer keep a lid on the flood of information pouring in from medical professionals and laypersons alike demonstrating that food is the answer to maintaining healthy, strong immune systems and living healthy lives. The proof is in the (sugar-free, gluten-free chia seed) pudding. People who exercise regularly, juice, and consume primarily a plant-based diet are slimmer than those who don't, and they have fewer occurrences of diabetes, heart disease, and cancer. They live longer, healthier, and have clearer skin. Most don't require walkers and wheelchairs to get around. They have more energy, feel and look younger, and are far less likely to require long-term medical and nursing care.

Death from fructose or pharmaceuticals or lack of exercise can be quick and unexpected or it can drone on and on as one hole-poking procedure after another slowly extinguishes your life one organ at a time. It doesn't have to be that way, though. If you want to avoid the pharmaceutical folly of today's high-tech medicine, it's up to you. Recognize that your daily habits have enormous impact on how you will die, and act accordingly. Take action while you still have time to prevent or reverse the ill state of health that has become commonplace. Read, research, experiment, and if you don't succeed on your own, get help. You are worth it, and so are those you love.

Bibliography

_____. 2005 Dietary Guidelines for Americans. Center for Nutrition Policy and Promotion, U.S. Department of Agriculture.

_____. World Cancer Research Fund, American Institute for Cancer Research. Food, Nutrition, Physical Activity, and the Prevention of Cancer: a Global Perspective. Washington DC: AICR, 2007.

American Diabetes Association website. http://www.diabetes.org.

American Medical Association website. http://www.ama-assn.org/ama.

Appel LJ, Moore TJ, Obarzanek E, et al. A clinical trial of the effects of dietary patterns on blood pressure. DASH Collaborative Research Group. N Engl J Med. 1997; 336:1117–24.

Appel LJ, Sacks FM, Carey VJ, et al. Effects of protein, monounsaturated fat, and carbohydrate intake on blood pressure and serum lipids:

results of the OmniHeart randomized trial. JAMA. 2005; 294:2455–64.

Blaylock, Russell L. Excitotoxins: The Taste That Kills. (Health Press, 1996).

Brechner, Arlene and Harold. Forty Something Forever: A Consumer's Guide to Chelation Therapy and Other Heart Savers. (Healthsavers Press, 1992).

Campbell, T. Colin, Thomas M. Campbell, et al. The China Study: The Most Comprehensive Study of Nutrition Ever Conducted and the Startling Implications for Diet, Weight Loss, and Long-Term Health. (BenBella Books, 2006).

Centers for Disease Control and Prevention website. http://www.cdc.gov.

Davis, William. Wheat Belly: Lose the Wheat, Lose the Weight, and Find Your Path Back to Health. (Rodale Press, Inc., 2011).

Dufty, William. Sugar Blues. (Grand Central Publishing, 1975).

Esselstyn CB Jr., Gendy G, Doyle J, Golubic M, Roizen MF. A way to reverse CAD? J Fam Pract. 2014;63:356-364b.

Fowler, Sharon P., et al. "Fueling the Obesity

Epidemic?" Obesity vol 16, no. 8 (2012); 1894–1900.

Fraser G, Katuli S, Anousheh R, Knutsen S, Herring P, Fan J. Vegetarian diets and cardiovascular risk factors in black members of the Adventist Health Study-2. Public Health Nutr. Published online March 17, 2014.

Giovannucci E, Liu Y, Platz EA, Stampfer MJ, Willett WC. Risk factors for prostate cancer incidence and progression in the Health Professionals Follow-up Study. Int J Cancer. 2007; 121:1571–78.

Gutiérrez OM, Muntner P, Rizk DV, et al. Dietary patterns and risk of death and progression to ESRD in individuals with CKD: a cohort study. Am J Kidney Dis. 2014;64:204-213.

He FJ, Nowson CA, Lucas M, MacGregor GA. Increased consumption of fruit and vegetables is related to a reduced risk of coronary heart disease: meta-analysis of cohort studies. J Hum Hypertens. 2007; 21:717–28.

He FJ, Nowson CA, MacGregor GA. Fruit and vegetable consumption and stroke: meta-analysis of cohort studies. Lancet. 2006; 367:320–26.
Hung HC, Joshipura KJ, Jiang R, et al. Fruit and vegetable intake and risk of major chronic disease. J Natl Cancer Inst. 2004; 96:1577–84.

Kavanaugh CJ, Trumbo PR, Ellwood KC. The U.S. Food and Drug Administration's evidence-based review for qualified health claims: tomatoes, lycopene, and cancer. J Natl Cancer Inst. 2007; 99:1074–85.

Kirk, Mimi. Live Raw: Food Recipes for Good Health and Timeless Beauty. (Skyhorse Publishing, 2011).

Kirk, Mimi. Live Raw Around the World: International Raw Food Recipes for Good Health and Timeless Beauty. (Skyhorse Publishing, 2013).

Kirschner, H. E. Live Food Juices: For Vim, Vigor, Vitality. (Kirschner Publications, 1957).

Mercola, Joseph. Sweet Misery: A Poisoned World, directed by J. T. Waldron (2006; Sound and Fury Productions, Inc.), DVD.

Ober, Clinton, Stephen T. Sinatra, and Martin Zucker. Earthing: The Most Important Health Discovery Ever? (Basic Health Publications, 2010).

Perlmutter, David and Kristin Loberg. Grain Brain: The Surprising Truth About Wheat, Carbs, and Suger—Your Brain's Silent Killers. (Little, Brown and Company, 2013).

Rosenthal, Joshua. Integrative Nutrition: Feed Your Hunger for Health & Happiness. (Integrative Nutrition Publishing, 2007).

Soret S, Mejia A, Batech M, Jaceldo-Siegl K, Harwatt H, Sabaté J. Climate change mitigation and health effects of varied dietary patterns in real-life settings throughout North America. Am J Clin Nutr. 2014;100:490S–495S.

Starfield, Barbara. "Is US Health Really the Best in the World?" JAMA vol 284, no. 4 (2000); 483–485.

Stoll, Andrew. The Omega-3 Connection: The Groundbreaking Anti-Depressant Diet and Brain Program. (Free Press, 2001).

Sugiyama T, Tsugawa Y, Tseng C, Kobayashi Y, Shapiro MF. Different time trends of caloric and fat intake between statin users and nonusers among US adults: gluttony in the time of statins? JAMA Intern Med. Published online April 24, 2014.

Telis, Gisela. "Can What You Eat Affect Your Mental Health?" The Washington Post, March 24, 2014.

United States Department of Agriculture website. usda.gov.

Wang X, Ouyang Y, Liu J, et al. Fruit and vegetable consumption and mortality from all causes, cardiovascular disease, and cancer: systematic review and dose-response meta-analysis of prospective cohort studies. BMJ. 2014;349:g4490.

Wendel, Brian. Forks Over Knives, directed by Lee Fulkerson (2011; Monica Beach Media), DVD.

Wikipedia website. www.wikipedia.org.

Wilson, James A. and Jonathan V. Wright. Adrenal Fatigue: The 21st-Century Stress Syndrome. (Smart Publications, 2001).

World Health Organization website. http://www.who.int.

16075289R00093

Made in the USA
San Bernardino, CA
17 October 2014